Healing STEPS

The A, B, C's Of Healing

DAVID H. BARDOWELL

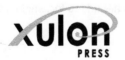

Table Of Contents

Introduction

$\mathcal{T}$he walls were dark brown, the kind of color you would see on an old 70's sitcom. The lights were dim, at least they seemed dim to me. As I sat waiting for my turn, it became clear this was not the type of place I ever thought I would be. The night before I had checked in to this hospital because there seemed like no other option. The place I found myself in was a place where other people went, not me. This place was a place for healing, a place for rehabilitation. We know it as Rehab!

Being a pastor, I find myself chuckling about my time in rehab. Heck, I could have become a famous reality T.V. star by starting a new show called, "Pastors in Rehab!" I'm sure many people would have tuned in! But that was then and this is now. I can laugh now because I am not in that dark place; there was no laughing back then. This was probably the darkest time of my life. That is saying a lot because my life was filled with many dark times, but this was the darkest of them all. I felt alone, scared, and uncomfortable. Little did I know, this was the beginning of my path to healing. This was the first step I needed to take. This place was exactly where I needed to be.

I think often of people who live with severe handicaps and illness; people who have chronic pain; people who have it much harder than me. How do they cope? I remember when my children were little. Our first two children were twins. I would find myself feeling sorry for myself because of how hard life was. What gave me perspective was seeing parents with triplets and quadruplets! I would wonder, "How do they do it?" Perspective is a good thing. I can look back at the dark times of my life and see with perspective how they helped move me along to where I am today. Those hard times were steps on a path to healing. They didn't seem so at the time, but as Johnny Nash sang, "I can see clearly now!"

I don't know where you are today. Maybe you are in a dark place. Maybe you know someone who is in a dark place. I can't tell you that I know how you feel, but I can tell you that I relate. I wish that I could sit around a table with you and a warm cup of coffee and each share about our experiences, pain, and victories. This is what I hope this book will accomplish. I hope that this book will give you hope. I hope that this book will help you see that there is a way out of your dark place; that your problems won't last forever. I know you probably don't feel that way right now, but I hope that as you read this book you will see the way out, you will see the steps that are right there before you to take.

Healing Steps is one way to experience healing, it is not the only way. There are many wonderful books and programs that can help you experience healing. I owe a lot to programs like AA, Celebrate Recovery, counselors, friends, and most of all God. I have gleaned from all of these, and each has influenced me on the path to healing. My goal in writing this book is to offer hope to you that healing can happen. The steps that I will talk about in this book have helped me and countless other people, and I know they can help you. I, in no way claim that these steps are magical or miraculous. They are suggested steps that will hopefully lead you to experience healing and peace as you walk them.

Healing steps, the A, B, C's of healing, is a way forward. Moving forward is the key to a successful, meaningful life. Feeling stuck, not being able to move forward causes anxiety and pain. We ask ourselves, "Will this ever end?" We start to wonder if the light at the end of the tunnel is really a train. After all, if you are anything like me, you've had your share of disappointments. I remember going to a motivational seminar, a seminar that was going to help me conquer the world. I spent hundreds of dollars and a tremendous amount of time only to come out feeling taken advantage of and ripped off. I also think of the many times I counted on someone or something to help me move forward only to feel betrayed and abandoned; they let me down. That is why I am here to tell you today that I can't promise that you will be healed, but I can promise you that you will see healing in the pages of this book because this book is my story, a story of healing. I will offer you hope, a hope that is everlasting, a hope that's found in God. I will show you some steps, steps that can move you forward from being stuck. Whatever your problem, you can find healing and victory. You can move forward and start living the life you were intended to live.

I also want to tell you that I am a Christian. I believe in Jesus Christ as my Lord and Savior. Therefore I am writing this book from a biblical, Christian point of view. My faith in Christ is more important to me than anything else. What God did for me is beyond explanation and comprehension. He is my way out. However, I also want you to know that faith without action is meaningless. If I don't walk what I believe then I cannot grow and I cannot heal. One of the most incredible gifts as a parent is to see your children take their first steps. I had the privilege and blessing to be present at each of my three children's first steps. I can still see them take those first steps, how wobbly they were, but before long they weren't just walking, they were running! Faith in God involves walking. We have to walk before we run. That is how we grow. So, I want to encourage you to walk. No matter if you believe in God or not, start to walk. The expert in anything was once a beginner. You won't be an expert at running if you don't begin by walking. That is how you will begin to move forward, walk. This is why I am writing this book. I want to help you walk.

In this book I will share stories, stories about myself and stories from the Bible. These stories are true. They really happened. My hope is from these stories you will find yourself able to relate to the characters in the story. Maybe you have already related to me being in rehab. Maybe you haven't been in rehab but you relate to feeling stuck, disappointed, betrayed. Maybe you understand the feeling of losing a loved one, feeling like you have lost everything. In 2004 I lost my father. That was the hardest thing I had ever experienced. Losing someone you love brings about all kinds of feelings and emotions. Some of the feelings are so strong they feel like they will take you down. Maybe you haven't lost someone to death, but maybe your child or children seem lost. Maybe your are losing your husband or your wife. You have tried everything to bring them back but nothing you do helps. In fact, they seem more distant than ever. Maybe you have a problem so big that you don't see any way out. There is a way out! I know you may not see it now, but don't give up. Your miracle may be just around the corner.

Dedication

Dedicated to my beautiful wife, Deborah, and my children, Austin, Ciera and Daniel, whom I love so very much.

Also dedicated to my church family at The Gate Christian Bible Church for their committed and faithful dedication and support. I cherish and value each one of you.

Most of all I dedicate this book to my Lord and Savior, Jesus Christ, whom without I would have no hope and no purpose. He is my healer.

Step 1: Admit

"How does one become a butterfly? They have to want to learn to fly so much that you are willing to give up being a caterpillar."
~Trina Paulus

"Blessed are the humble, for theirs is the kingdom of heaven" –
Jesus Christ

There I was, sitting in rehab, depressed, discouraged, and hopeless. My father had died one year earlier, and I had fallen into a deep depression. My anxiety went through the roof; I couldn't sleep or eat. Things were not looking very good for me. I wondered what in the world was going on? I would hear of people who came to these places. I always thought that they were weak; that they needed to just snap out of it. At least that was what I believed; but now I was the weak one, and I couldn't snap out of it.

My father and I were close. He was a strong, self-willed man who at the age of thirteen went to work and took care of his six brothers and one sister. His mother had passed away and his father was pretty much AWOL. I always respected my father's strength. I remember him sharing a story with me about his strength and will power. When he was young, he smoked 6 packs of cigarettes a day! Then one day he just quit. I asked him how he quit, and he said, "willpower!" I wanted to be like my dad. He was strong. I always felt that I had to be the strong one. Even as a young child, I sensed the world around me was crumbling, my family was falling apart, and for some reason I felt responsible. Since I was the oldest child, I felt like I had to hold it together. It's hard to hold it together for very long. After my dad died, I couldn't hold it together any longer, so I fell apart.

There's a story of a father whose wife left the house for some errands. She asked him to watch their little boy. The father came up with a great idea. Since he was very tired, he gave his son a project. He noticed a picture of a globe in the newspaper. He ripped up the newspaper into little pieces and asked his son to put the "world" back together. The father laid down on the couch for what he thought would be a long nap. In just a few minutes, however, the son finished his assignment and said with a smile on his face, "Dad, I'm finished!" To his father's amazement, his son had put the globe in the newspaper back together perfectly. "How did you do this so quickly, son?" the father asked. "Dad," the son said with glee in his heart, "there was a picture of a person on the other side. When I put my person back together, the world looked a lot better!" Putting a person back together is hard work. It took an entire regiment of horses and king's men to put Humpty Dumpty back together. I was falling apart, just like him.

We All Need To Sleep And Eat!

It started out with not being able to sleep. I would spend entire nights being awake, thinking about my father and how much he suffered. It didn't make sense. Why would such a strong man suffer like that? I felt cheated and angry. My father was too young to suffer and die such a painful death. He struggled many years with diabetes, which took his leg and his life at the age of seventy-six. I missed my father so much. The pain built up in me like no other pain. I had never gone through losing a loved one, so this was all new to me. I was the first one to keep working, keep living, no matter what pain I had, but this pain was different. It was a deep emotional pain, felt way down even into my bones. The pain was so strong that I didn't want to eat. When I did eat, I felt sick. I must say, being from a Middle-Eastern, South American, born-in-Jamaica background, eating was part of my personality! I loved to eat. Now I couldn't even do what I loved to do. I felt so confused and anxious. I had always been an anxious person. As a child I would bite my nails, and I had struggled with bodily twitches. Now it was as if the anxiety had nowhere to go, so it started coming out all over the place like a sewage spill. Not being able to sleep and eat was bad enough, but now I was not even able to think straight. I couldn't sleep or work. I seriously felt like I was "losing it".

At the advice of some friends and family, I went to see a doctor. The doctor suggested that I take some pills, anti-depressants. No way was I going to take an anti-depressant! Those were for weak people! I was strong, like my dad. I could get through this. But after months of dealing with constant anxiety, which moved to panic attacks, and weeks of not sleeping, I decided to try them. If you've ever taken anti-depressants, you will agree with me that they are some of the hardest pills to take—at first. The side effects are horrendous! They actually made me feel worse. So, knowing this, the doctor gave me some other pills, pills to help me sleep and relax. These pills were only to be taken for a short while until the anti-depressants kicked in. The pills the doctor gave me are known as benzodiazepines. You may know them as sedatives or sleeping pills. The first time I took that pill, I felt great! It reminded me of the sixteen years from the age of thirteen to twenty-nine that I spent drinking and taking drugs. Taking those pills helped me sleep and eat, and I was a happy camper. But the happiness didn't last long.

One thing that every drug addict knows is that drugs will eventually wear off and you will need more. Because of my past experience with drug and alcohol abuse, I knew that I would have to take more of the "benzos" to get the same effect as when I took less. I was very careful. I would cut the pills in half to make sure that I only took the amount I needed. But I knew that I was becoming dependent on them when I would think about the next pill, and the next pill. I would count each pill and would make sure that I order refills before I ran out. I thought of the pill as a solution rather than a remedy. The pill became my solace and refuge. As like any pill, drink, or drug, they wear off and eventually start to cause the same effect as they were prescribed to treat. For instance, drinking or smoking pot will help someone feel relaxed at first, but if the person keeps using these vices, they will eventually cause anxiety because the body will crave more. Now, I'm not saying that everyone will experience this, but I did. I'm not sure if it has something to do with the way I'm wired, but the pill that used to help with anxiety and panic attacks started backfiring and causing more anxiety and panic attacks. Now, on top of everything else, I was a pill addict!

It was then that I realized I needed to rely on my strong will. I needed my willpower to kick in. After all, my dad quit smoking by his will; why couldn't I quit these pills by *my* will? I started to cut back. At first I was fine, but then everything went haywire. At the same time that I was trying to stop the pills, I developed a painful infection that would not go away. This lasted for weeks. The pain was so bad that I had a hard time sleeping, and I couldn't function the way I was used to functioning. The anxiety and panic attacks got worse, and the pain became unbearable. However, I was not going to let this get to me, so I became more defiant and stronger-willed.

Have you ever seen a battleship? When I was young, we used to visit the San Diego harbor. My friend's dad was a Navy veteran, and he used to take us to see the ships. Battleships are incredibly well built and strong! But the thing about battleships is that they take forever to turn around. It takes an average of fifty miles for a battleship to turn around. That's the problem with being so strong-willed. It takes forever to turn around.

There's a story of a battleship and a lighthouse. It was night, and the battleship was at sea. Off in the distance the captain of the battleship saw a light heading towards him. He immediately got on his radio and told the light to move course for he was going straight towards a battleship. The light answered back, "You change course". The captain couldn't believe what he was hearing, so he sent back another message. "I'm a battleship. I demand you change course", to which the light answered back "I'm a lighthouse, you better change course." The battleship was heading straight into a lighthouse and didn't know it. I was heading straight into a lighthouse and was not going to budge. That is until October 25, 2005. That was the day I entered rehab.

Dark Times at Rehab High

I remember seeing the movie, "Fast Times at Ridgemont High". The movie was about the "fun" we all had in high school – sex, drugs, and rock and roll. Those times may be fun at first, but every decision has a consequence. Even though I was on a new path with God, the decisions I made early on in life were catching up to me. Every decision has a consequence. The consequence can be good and healthy or not good and not healthy. For me, the decisions I made as a young man were finally coming to a head, and I was running out of willpower.

The morning I asked my wife to take me to the hospital was a Monday. It was just like any other morning I had experienced over the past year. I didn't sleep much the night before, my anxiety level was out the roof, and the panic attacks were happening multiple times a day and night. The day prior, I had taught one of our leadership classes at church and barely got through the class. No one would have noticed because I was really good at hiding pain! The pain from my infection was not diminishing, and my will had run out. The medicine was not working, and I was to the point of either finding help or ending my life. I say this with respect, not flippantly. I literally was at the end of my rope. I felt horrible for feeling this way. Me, a Christian man, a pastor, someone who taught about God's incredible faithfulness and power, was actually thinking about ending my life. I've heard people say that those thoughts are selfish thoughts. What about my wife, my kids, my church? I understand where people who say that are coming from, but the people who say that do not understand how incredibly powerful those thoughts can be. For someone to get to the point of thinking those thoughts, it comes from living day-after-day not seeing any hope of things turning around, and the light at the end of the tunnel IS a train coming straight towards you. If anyone should have been able to snap out of it, it should have been me, but the only thing that snapped was my will to live.

"Deborah," I said with a soft, ashamed voice, "I need you to take me to the hospital." Imagine the humiliation I felt saying those words to my wife. After all, I am her husband, the man she married who promised to take care of her, to be strong. Now I was asking her to take care of me. I know for some people that doesn't seem like a big deal, but for someone who was taught to never show weakness, never give up, and always stand strong, it was a huge deal. Nevertheless, there was no other choice. Either I would receive help or I would die.

Hospitals Can Be Helpful

Once checked into rehab, I waited in line to see the psychiatrist. There were so many other people there with me; it seemed for a moment I was in the wrong place. So many people needed help. I guess I underestimated the depth of pain in the world. I was just like them and didn't even know it. Deborah had taken me as far as she could go. The people in charge searched me and asked me to drop all my possessions—cell phone, wallet, and pills, in a bin. They promised they would return those things to me once I checked out. Heck, they also asked for my shoelaces! It took me a while to figure that one out. I guess when someone wants to end their life, they will use any means to accomplish it. Out of all my possessions, the pills were the hardest to turn over to them. I really had come to a point of severe dependency. Either this hospital would help or the pills would help. The pills had stopped helping, so now it was up to the hospital. "Please, God, help me!"

The psychiatrist was surprised at the low dosage of anti-depressant I was taking. I told him that I didn't like the way they made me feel. He spoke with a clear, sergeant kind of voice, "That doesn't matter right now! You either take more dosage and feel better or stay the way you are." You know, I had always had a mistrust of doctors. I don't know why. I think it was just because I am a stubborn person. I don't like people telling me what to do or how to do it. But at that precise moment, I decided to do what the doctor said. I guess being in a place like this meant that I was serious about getting help. The doctor raised my prescription so much that the next few nights were worse than the other nights. Plus, add the fact that I was now totally off the other medication. I felt like I was having out of body experiences!

Nurses Can Be Angels

The second day in the hospital I found myself walking around in total disarray and confusion. I didn't know what to do or where to go. That's when I saw her ... a lady with a smile, wearing a nurse outfit. My first thought was, "why would anyone smile in a place like this?" She smiled and said to me "You need to go into that room there." Her voice sounded distorted and shaky, like someone playing a role in the Twilight Zone. It seemed like I was in a dream. I had decided that since my plan wasn't working, I was going to listen to the doctors and the nurses! So, I found myself opening the door to the designated room and sitting in a chair. Only one or two other people were in the room with me. I felt alone and scared. Why am I here? By the way, I never did see that nurse again.

A Sign

As I looked around, I saw a sign on the wall. The sign was a simple sign, white with black letters. As I looked at the sign, I noticed that it was not like the other signs I saw in the hospital. On those signs were notated things that I could not do. This sign was different because it contained a list of things I *should* do. Each thing had a number assigned to it. There were twelve numbered items. I looked closer to discover that these numbers were indicative of certain steps someone should take, kind of like the Ten Commandments.

Have you ever felt like the light bulb came on? My wife, Deborah, and I have been married now for twenty-two years. When I met my wife, I had a moment of clarity when the light bulb came on. The moment of clarity was this, "David, you should marry her because you will never meet anyone more beautiful inside and out than her." That was a moment of clarity when I knew I was making the right decision. Those moments don't seem to come often enough, yet are so freeing. Well, my moment of clarity was written on the wall! As I stared at that sign, it was as if the fog lifted just long enough for me to read step one with clarity:

Step 1 (of the 12 Steps of Alcoholics Anonymous): We admitted we were powerless over our addiction and that our lives had become unmanageable.

The sign I was looking at was a list of the 12 steps of Alcoholics Anonymous. I had heard of them, but really never paid any attention to them until now. The moment of clarity stayed long enough for me to focus on one very important word: **Admit**. "We admitted we were powerless." The rest of the class was a blur, but the moment of clarity stuck with me the rest of my day, week, and now life. If you are familiar with the twelve steps, you know that each step moves to the next step. In other words, you can't take step twelve without taking step one. I just kept staring at number one.

Do you hate standing in line as much as I? I love Disneyland. It was one of my favorite places to go when I was young, but I hated waiting in line. I would figure out ways to move to the front of the line so as to not have to wait an hour for a ride. I think this is an example of human nature. We hate to wait. As the great theologian Tom Petty said, "The waiting is the hardest part."[1] The problem with impatience is that often times we miss something foundational, a lesson, a blessing, because we move ahead too fast. When baking a cake, it is important to follow instructions so the cake will hold together. It is the same with these steps. You can't skip a step; you have to start with step one.

This is where my story takes a turn. The battle ship started doing a 180! Up to this point, I had thought that I had power over my problem. I was like MacGyver, the guy in the old T.V. show; I could find a way out of any perilous situation. I thought that I was indestructible, that I could carry the weight of the world on my shoulders. Now, sitting in this room, in rehab, in a gown with all my possessions taken away, I realized that I am not as strong as I think I am. I skipped step one because I never thought that I needed to admit anything, yet alone admit my need for help.

Why can't I admit I am wrong? That was the question I asked myself after every time I had an argument with my wife. I knew I was wrong, but something got in the way of me admitting it. That something is the Greek word "ego" which means "I." I stand in the way of admitting I am wrong and need help. No one can stop me from saying I am wrong; it is "I" who stops me from admitting I am wrong. Have you ever felt like that? Has your ego gotten in the way of your own admission? Well, you are not alone. Many people struggle with admitting being wrong, that they might need help. It sometimes takes a trip to the hospital to admit your need for help.

The Problem with Problems

I want to make something clear, and it is the premise of this entire book. My problem was not with the pills; my problem was deeper than that. You will see the depth of my problem as this book unfolds. Therefore, just because step one to an alcoholic, or a drug addict, or anybody with a problem, may deal with admitting their addiction, what you are really admitting is that you have a problem. The problems with problems are that often times they just don't go away. The problem may be big or small, short or long, but nevertheless it is still a problem. That is why this book deals with helping you with your problems. Your problem may be different than mine. Maybe you don't have a problem with pills; maybe your problem didn't end you up in rehab. Maybe your problem has to do with your marriage, your finances, your health, your family, your kids. Taking steps toward healing begins with admitting you have a problem. Therefore, the steps in this book, the A, B, C's of healing, don't just deal with addictions, they deal with problems:

Healing Step 1: **Admit** I have a problem that I can't solve on my own.

Step 1 is admitting that you have a problem, a problem that you can't solve on your own. You admit that the problem is problematic and is causing more problems. The problem may be major or minor. Nevertheless, you admit that the only way to get rid of this problem is by getting help. As I sat in that chair staring at the wall, I noticed that I skipped step one. I began with step **2**, "**Believe** that God can solve my problem and give me the help I need." Believing is extremely important to being healed, but like baking a cake, you can't skip steps. Why was my life falling apart? Why did I not have a strong foundation? It was not due to my unbelief; it was due to my unwillingness to admit.

My Friend Bart

Bart was blind, blind as a bat. He could not afford glasses, so he relied on his friends to help him move around town. Bart had been blind since birth, so he did not have any idea what seeing looked like. Bart dreamed of the day he could see, and he promised that if that day ever came, it would be the best day of his life. His friends, however, had little hope because healing a blind man, especially a man blind from birth, was unheard of.

I remember Bart's day of healing like it was yesterday. The town was bustling, it was a workday, and everyone was busy. Bart, with the help of his friends, was going to the grocery store to buy food. All of a sudden, the people in the town began moving quickly to the town square. We all wondered what was going on. When I asked someone, he answered, "Haven't you heard? There's a miracle-worker in town, and He is looking for people to heal!" I looked at Bart, whose ears, by the way, were like elephant's! He heard every word the gentleman said. I took his hand and walked as fast as we could. Bart fell down along the way sometimes, but got back up. He was so excited about hopefully meeting this miracle-worker.

When we got to the town square, it was packed! People were gathered all around, and the miracle-worker was inundated with requests. We were asked to stand back, that the miracle-worker was not going to be seeing anyone else that day. That's when Bart began to pray. He prayed so hard that I could hear him over the crowd saying, "God, if you're real, please show me, please heal me". There's something about an honest, sincere prayer that gets people's attention. Well, it must have gotten the miracle-worker's attention, because out of the blue he called on Bart. "Bart (how did he know his name?), come up here." A hush fell over the crowd. Bart tried to maneuver himself through the dense crowd, falling over people along the way. Some people laughed and mocked him, "He doesn't have time for you!" they shouted. Everyone could tell Bart was blind, that's why the question the miracle-worker was about to ask him was so strange. When Bart finally made it to the stage, the attendants helped him up. Once on the stage, they introduced him to the miracle-worker, who shook Bart's hand. The miracle-worker took a moment and then asked a question that seemed to echo into the depth of his soul. It was a kind of question that seemed almost holy, or somewhat eternal. He asked, "Bart, what do you want me to do for you?"

Now, I must say, being in that crowd that day was an amazing experience. Seeing all those people coming to be healed. One after the other, the miracle-worker healed them, and not once did I hear him ask the question he asked Bart. For some reason, though, he decided to ask his question of Bart. Later it made sense why he asked, but at this moment it was confusing and brought tension into Bart's heart. The crowd began to jostle and laugh. They didn't believe that Bart could be healed.

I want to take a short break from this story and explain something to you. There are lots of people who have problems who are comfortable in their problems. It is almost as if their problem has become a part of them; and if their problem were to leave, they would lose their identity. The elephant in the room is their problem. Their problem might not be an addiction, but soon enough, if they don't deal with their problem, their problem will deal with them. That's when the problem could take over and get the best of them. It could even become an addiction. In other words, for some reason, their identity is wrapped up in their problem. I believe that some people would rather keep living the same discouraging, disillusioned, confusing life rather than be healed and live a healed, productive, fulfilling, focused life. I don't know why this is. Maybe it is because they are afraid that the other side of healing is scary. Maybe it's because their problem, even though destructive, is so engrained in their life that they would rather die than change. I don't know, but this is the reality for some people. This was not the case for Bart.

Bart, standing before the miracle-worker, could not believe his chance had come. "Would the miracle-worker really be able to make me see?" At first, Bart may have felt unsure of the miracle-worker's credentials, since he failed to see what everyone else knew as plain as day, Bart was blind. But that faded away when he realized that his opportunity to be healed was upon him. So, even in the midst of mocking and laughter, Bart summoned up the courage to say, "I want to see!" The words still echo in my soul today, four powerful yet simple words spoken from a sincere heart. I guess that was enough to move the miracle-worker to work in Bart's life. For in what seemed like only a second of time, the miracle-worker spoke with conviction saying, "Go…your faith has healed you." In that instance, Bart started living in a whole new world. He opened his eyes, and for the first time saw his friends, his family, the trees, and the sky. Everything was new to him, like a child playing in fresh-fallen snow. Bart was a new person. What was once a caterpillar was now a butterfly. His problem was gone, and he walked home with dignity.

I must make an admission. This story is not actually my story, and I was not there. This story is in the Bible, in Mark chapter ten. Bart's name is actually Bartimaeus, which means "honorable son." Bart was not very honorable in his blindness, but that is the amazing thing about God ...He looks beyond from where you are to who you can be. Bart may not have been honorable to the crowd, but he was honorable to God. Every person has dignity because the Bible says that we are all made in God's image. But because of sin, sickness, and pain, the world is filled with problems. Problems, however, are a platform for God to perform miracles. Some people are blind, not physically blind, but spiritually blind. They don't want their eyes to be opened. They would rather just live in the darkness of their problem, because if their eyes were opened, they may see their need for God. God solved Bart's problem, and he can solve your problem too!

Admit

Why did Jesus ask Bart the question, "What do you want me to do?"–was it because Jesus didn't know he was blind? Of course not! Jesus knew Bart was blind; he was just waiting for Bart to admit his blindness. Healing Steps, the A, B, C's of healing, begins with the letter "A." "**A**" means Admit, admitting I have a problem of which I can't solve. Being blind is a huge problem. Even today, medicine has a hard time dealing with blindness. To God, however, it is just a problem. I say "just" a problem, not to diminish the problem, but to elevate God. God can do anything He wants at anytime He wants to do it. Jesus Christ decided that it was good to heal old Bart. But I don't want you to miss a very important part of the story. <u>God's part was to heal, Bart's part was to admit;</u> admit he had a problem. The fact that Jesus asked Bart, "What do you want me to do for you?" shows that Jesus was interested in hearing that Bart was in a place of humility, a place of admission. Do you think that Jesus needed to hear about Bart's need? If so, then Jesus is not God. I believe in a God who knows everything, therefore it was not that Jesus had to find out what Bart needed, it was that Jesus wanted Bart to know what Bart needed. Admitting is not for God's sake it, is for your sake. God already knows what you need. He is just waiting for you to humble yourself enough to ask for help. Until I can get to the point of admission, I cannot get to the point of healing. I must admit my need for help because it is in that admission that I hear my own voice saying "This is too big for me to handle." That is where the healing begins.

At this point I would encourage you to seriously consider your life in regards to your problems and in regards to healing. What needs to be admitted? Maybe you need to admit that you are like a battleship heading straight for a lighthouse. Maybe your admission needs to deal with your stubbornness. I was stubborn in not listening to doctors, not taking advice, trying to run my life without any input from others. Maybe you need to admit that, like me, you are not as strong as you think you are. Willpower runs out, God's power is limitless. Whatever your admission, remember that healing begins the moment you can <u>"Admit you have a problem that you can't solve on your own.</u> Bart could admit that his problem was bigger than he could solve because he was blind. There was no way, outside of a miracle, that he would ever see. The problem is that, like Bart, we are blind, not physically blind, but still blind. We are blind to our problems, blind to our need for help. We would rather go through life letting our problems run the show rather than letting someone who can solve our problem take the stage and do a miracle! Why would you not admit your need for help? Let me ask you a question. Looking at your life today, would you say that your life is what you want it to be? If not, then why not admit that? Say it openly, out loud, "I need help!" Those three words can change your life.

I invite you to take this first step, step 1. All you have to do is "Admit." You don't even have to "Believe" because that is step 2. Begin with step 1. You can just say out loud:

"I need help. I am struggling with a problem (name your problems here if you know them). I can't handle this/these problems. I need someone or something stronger than me to deal with them. I realize that I can't solve my own problem on my own, because I am not as strong as I think I am. I have tried for too long to carry the weight of the world on my shoulders. I am tired and I need help. God, if you're real, please help me."

As I mentioned at the beginning of this book, I can't promise you that your problem will go away, but I can promise you that you will see a way out. You don't have to be in that dark place for the rest of your life. You can have peace, you can have joy, and most of all you can be healed!

Step 2: Believe

"To one who has faith, no explanation is necessary. To one without faith, no explanation is possible."–Thomas Aquinas

"If you believe you will receive... whatever you ask for...."
– Jesus Christ (Matthew 21:22)

I was born on the Caribbean island of Jamaica in 1962. My father was born there also; my mother is from Colombia, South America. In 1966 we moved to Southern California, and it is there where I grew up. At the age of six, my mother signed me up for music lessons, accordion lessons to be exact. I was so young, and my fingers so small, that the teacher suggested the smaller keys of the accordion rather than the piano. Thank God, however, that my hands grew, because accordion was not going to be my ticket to anywhere!

I loved music. When I discovered music, my life changed. All of a sudden, I felt like I was uniquely important. My family life growing up was shaky to say the least; music helped bring a sense of security into my life. Lack of trust and lack of boundaries caused a lot of stress and anxiety, which led to a constant sense of fear that everything would eventually fall apart. I had to fight to be my own person.

This is why music became so important to me. Music let me be my own person. I felt even more like my own person when I wrote my first song for my fourth grade teacher. I was eight years old. I didn't just write it in my head, I actually wrote the notes out on manuscript paper by hand. That's pretty impressive for an eight year old! It was almost ten years later when I wrote my second song, a song written for a friend who died on the operating table. It was the first time I wrote a song out of sadness, but it wouldn't be the last. Music was my way of communicating how I felt, which most of the time was discouragement and sadness.

At the age of twelve, while attending junior high school, my life changed again. While on an honor choir tour to San Diego, I met a drummer who became my best friend. His name is John Stamos. John went on to have a very successful career in T.V. When I met John, we were just two kids who wanted to play music. I recruited John as my drummer. He, along with my very talented brother Philip, began to rehearse in my parent's living room. We soon built up enough of a repertoire to start playing gigs. Our first gig was at John's uncle's house. We were hired to play music for three hours, from 8pm to 11pm. We were so excited! But then it hit me; we only knew five songs! That wasn't even a half-hour's worth of music! Boy, how life is less complicated when you're a kid. We showed up for the gig, set up our instruments and began to play. The people were already pretty drunk by the time we started playing. Little did I know that John's father had turned the clock forward two hours, so instead of us starting at 8pm, we were starting at 10pm; well, at least that was according to the new time that was set by John's dad. No one even noticed that we only played for around forty-five minutes!

Life was so fun playing music together. Music was what I lived for; that was until I discovered other things. I discovered alcohol at the age of thirteen. What I loved about alcohol was how it made me feel. It took away my shyness and gave me courage. I was so shy, so anxious. I was stuck in the prison of insecurity and shame. Alcohol was my ticket out of being stuck, or so I thought. Shortly after discovering alcohol, I discovered marijuana. That was even better because the good feelings lasted longer! It was around this time that I also discovered girls. My first intimate relation with a girl was horrendous. It was not like what I expected it to be. This girl was not a girl at all... she was a grown woman. I don't think I have words to explain how I felt after that first experience. I could say it felt good, but I would be lying. It felt terribly wrong. I was just a boy. I felt taken advantage of, ripped off, ashamed. I struggle writing this because I'm sure some people will not understand how a young boy would feel ripped off by having sex. I believe there are certain ages in a person's life when they are supposed to experience certain things. Sex is something that should be experienced with the person you will spend the rest of your life with, not when you're 15 years old and the other person is 20-something. This experience tainted my view of sex and opened up the door to many other sexual encounters that helped taint this sacred act even more. Nevertheless, even though I felt ashamed, I just swept it under the rug and tried to drink my feelings away. So many other things happened in my life that were "not supposed to happen," that I just checked it off as another "not supposed to happen" moment.

My life was now engrossed with three things: Alcohol, Drugs, and Women. I was a full-fledged musician! I continued my pursuit of becoming a better musician by attending college and receiving a Bachelor of Music Degree. While in college, I received a phone call from an alumnus of the college I was attending. His name is Richard Carpenter. Richard and his sister Karen, and their band, "The Carpenters," changed the landscape of pop music with some of the most beautiful songs and arrangements ever recorded. Richard asked me if I would join him on a concert tour to Japan. That was my first taste of professional music touring, and I loved it! I fell in love with travelling and couldn't wait to travel more. Over the next few years, I had the privilege of touring the world with some well-known recording artists, notably, surf band "Jan and Dean", and Mike Love of "The Beach Boys." I think back now to the incredible experiences I had touring with such famous bands. Sadly, however, I can also think back to how miserable I was. No matter what stage I was on, where I was playing, or whom I was playing with, I was miserable. I felt empty. There was a hole in my heart that couldn't be filled. The alcohol and drugs were not working like they used to, and the music was getting monotonous. It was also around this time that I really got turned on to the band, "The Doors", especially the lead singer Jim Morrison. I actually got to record in the Door's drummer's recording studio, which as you would expect, if you know anything about that band, had everything I wanted in a recording studio, mostly the right drugs! Jim Morrison was a free spirit; it seemed like he was not bound to anyone or anything. I admired him, but Jim killed himself. I wanted to be like Jim. I was not happy, always angry, and never content. I hated the way I felt and tried to self-medicate so I wouldn't feel my feelings anymore, but nothing was working. I just wanted it all to end. The things I thought would make me happy and give me fulfillment were letting me down. Everyone else abandoned me, and now the three things I loved the most–alcohol, drugs, and women, were doing the same.

<u>Bike Rides Are Helpful</u>

I have a deep love for the ocean, so I decided to move into a house with some friends only a few miles from my favorite beach. One day while riding my bike to the beach, I prayed a prayer, a prayer that would change my life. Before I share my prayer, I must share my religious experience because like the other three: alcohol, drugs and women, religion let me down too.

Every Sunday as a child, my parents would wake us up to go to church. We would get in the car and drive over forty miles to attend church. This was a place that was very important to my parents, but to be honest with you, I never wanted to go. That is until I discovered that I could play music at church! Then church became one of my favorite places. You know, it's weird to think of church as another thing I could receive something from rather than a place where I could give, but church was never about giving, it was always about getting. I could prove to people that I was important and valuable by how well I played music. I could receive the "pat on the backs" that I thought I deserved, which helped me feel important. I could prove to God that I was important and valuable by how many times I would attend church and how much time I would give him in my schedule. I felt like he would keep track of these things, and that he would love me in return.

One day, however, we got the word that the new priest was going to get rid of the band at church and just allow organ and singing. When I asked the priest why he was doing this, he said, "Because that's the way it's always been done." That answer let me down; it changed my view of church and of God. Although I didn't love God and I didn't love church, at least I loved the reason I went to church…

music. Now that reason was taken away. Something that I trusted, something that gave me fulfillment, was gone, just like everything else. It is one thing to feel like people let you down, but it's totally another thing to feel like God let you down. That's how I felt, and I was angry. Plus, I thought God was angry with me, so we had a great thing going!

Now... back to my bike ride. It was a sunny day, and I decided to ride to the beach. While riding, I prayed a prayer. This prayer truly changed my life. It wasn't some sanctimonious, long prayer. It was a short, simple prayer, "<u>God, if you're real, please show me</u>." I don't know where that prayer came from. After all, God and I were not very tight. I guess it just came from my heart. The pain and hurt had, up until this point, masked this prayer. But for some reason, that day, it was unmasked as it came forth like the sun in the western sky. After my prayer, I finished my ride to the beach, walked around, thought about my empty life, looked at the sea, the sky, and then rode back home. Nothing changed, at least not right away.

<u>Wrong Numbers Can Change Your Life</u>!

Have you ever received a phone call that changed your life? I had always hoped I would get a call from Ed McMahon telling me I had won the Publishers Clearing House lottery! That call never came. However, a call did come that was better than any prize.

The phone call I am about to describe is worth much more than a million dollars because it changed my life from the inside out.

The day my life started to really change began like any other. I started my day getting ready to teach at the high school where I worked, a job I did, not because I loved it, but because it paid my bills.

While getting ready for work, my phone rang. I answered the phone to hear the voice on the other end ask "Is Bob there?" "You have the wrong number", I replied, to which he responded, "Jesus loves you."

I can't wait to find out one day who that person was who called me. Maybe in heaven, I will meet him. For now, let's just say that those three simple words, *"Jesus loves you"* were my ticket out of the hell in which I lived. After hanging up the phone, I thought about what that man said. "Jesus loves me?" That can't be true. What about all the bad things I did? What about all the bad thoughts I've had? What about my anger towards him? I'm sure he was angry with me too. Jesus was always with me, if only on my wall. I always had with me a crucifix, and on the crucifix was Jesus. As long as Jesus stayed on the crucifix, everything would be okay. I think I thought that if I had Jesus with me on the cross, then he would protect me, so no matter where I lived, the first thing I would do was take the crucifix out of my suitcase and hang it on my wall. The words, "Jesus loves you," especially when received from a misdialed phone call, did not match the Jesus I knew. There he was, on my wall. I looked at him and thought, "There is no way you could ever love me." I wasn't ready to believe those words. That is until the next day, and the day after that.

Good Things Come In Threes

My mom used to tell me that people die in threes. When I would hear of someone famous dying, I would wait to find out who the other two would be. That is a pretty morbid way to think, but most of the time she was right! Well, I believe that good things come in three. Here's why: The day after the misdialed phone call, I was shopping in a mall. Malls in Southern California are always filled with people. One person in this mall stood out. He was sitting on a bench in front of a store. He looked rather serious, serious enough for me not to want to make eye contact. I tried to look away but he was staring right at me. At that moment, time seemed to slow down; it was like a slow motion movie. Everyone else in the mall disappeared, and it was only he and I. He looked at me, and me at him. His mouth opened, and he said "Hey man," followed by those three simple words, *"Jesus loves you."* At that moment, time sped up, I looked back, and he was gone.

Have you ever watched a movie more than once? There are some movies that I can watch over and over and not get bored. One of those movies is "Taken." There is something about that movie, that even though I know the ending, the movie still captivates me. The misdialed phone call and the man in the mall are kind of like a movie. It is a movie that I keep playing over and over in my head. Even though I know the ending, it still captivates me. Why does it captivate me? It captivates me because the ending is so good.

As I said earlier, good things come in three. Even though I had heard "Jesus loves you," said to me twice, it wasn't until the third time when the message really sank in and made sense. Roughly a week after seeing the man on the bench in the mall, I found myself wandering around a crowded parking lot trying to find my car. Back then we didn't have remote control remotes to help us find our cars with beeping sounds, so sometimes it was a tedious job finding where I had parked. While searching for my car, I noticed another car. This car stood out. It was a pink V.W. bug. V.W. bugs stand out enough, but this one was pink! It wasn't the color of the car that caught my attention; it was what was written on the car. Written on the car, in bright fluorescent paint were these three simple words… you guessed it, *"Jesus loves you."*

One of my favorite cartoon shows is "SpongeBob Square Pants." I love SpongeBob because he is so upbeat. My favorite character in that cartoon, however, is Patrick. Patrick is a starfish with no brains. Patrick talks like he has no brains, he stutters and drools. One of my favorite episodes is the one where the cartoonist shows us the inside of Patrick's head. It was an episode where Patrick all of a sudden became smart. In order to show Patrick's brain starting to function, the cartoonist used a windmill. The windmill in his brain all of a sudden started working, and he became smarter and smarter as the windmill worked faster and faster. That's what happened to me that day, my windmill started working! After hearing the guy on the other end of the phone say, *"Jesus loves you,"* and after seeing the man in the mall who said, *"Jesus loves you,"* it was the third time, seeing *"Jesus loves you"* on that car that finally sank in! I got it! Good things come in threes.

I don't know why it took three times for me to get it. Maybe I'm like Patrick. Or maybe I'm like Peter in the Bible. Jesus had to show Peter three times that he loved him. Jesus had to show me the same. Like Peter, I never felt loved by anyone. Allowing myself to be loved was too risky because usually the person I would love would abandon me or let me down. At least that is how I experienced love up until this point. I really never had a problem with feeling and expressing love towards someone else. It was the accepting love that was most difficult. I never felt worthy of being loved, and I never trusted that their love for me would last. Jesus went out of his way to tell me that he loved me – three times! It took three times for me to accept his love for me. After seeing the car, I remembered my prayer, "God, if you're real, please show me," and he did!

I don't know where you are with God. Maybe you have had a bad experience, or like me, would never feel worthy of God's love. The truth is–none of us are worthy! That is why it is called grace. Grace comes from the Greek word "charis," which is unmerited favor. Grace is a free gift; you can't earn it. When someone is gracious it is not because of what we have done for them, it is because of how they choose to treat us. God is gracious towards those who humbly call on him for help. I need this kind of help – grace. You may think of grace as something for weak people, I think it is for those who are strong enough to admit their need for help. I didn't plan the things that happened in my life to lead me to God, God planned them, by his grace. I was like an actor just playing my part, which was the part of believing. God did everything else. Believe me, I could have never saved myself. God is the only one who can save me. God freely offers his love to anyone who will accept it. For me, it took a series of events for me to understand that God loves me. Once I did, my life forever changed.

Here's the Good News: Jesus doesn't just love me; He loves everyone – *"For God so loved the world that whoever believes in him will not perish but have everlasting life"* (John 3:16). Are you part of this world? Then God loves you! I know this may seem so foreign and absurd that the God of the universe would love you, but it's true! You may ask, "What about all the bad things I have done?" "What about all the bad thoughts I've had?" Let me tell you something, no one is perfect. God knows I'm not perfect. Jesus said that He came to love sinners. I sinned against God many times, but He still chose to love me. Do I deserve this love? Certainly not! That is why it is such an amazing kind of love. Think of this chapter as a phone call, a phone call that you can answer if you would only believe.

Peter

Most people, even if they are not Christians or churchgoers, know about Peter. Peter was one of Jesus' best friends, a disciple. They met one day on the beach. Peter was working on his boat, and Jesus called his name. Jesus loved Peter, but Peter did not accept God's love at first. Peter was afraid of God. He thought God was mad at him. Most men of Peter's age would be following a rabbi, a teacher by now. The fact that Peter was working on his boat shows that either Peter was not interested in following God, or that no rabbi was interested in Peter. But this day was different. Jesus called Peter's name, and Peter answered. Even though Peter seemed content on the outside, he was not happy on the inside. Peter was fishing for something that he couldn't find in the lake, and Jesus knew exactly what he needed. Peter was an actor in God's movie and was about to have a life changing experience with God.

The Love Boat

One of my favorite T.V. shows growing up was "The Love Boat." I made sure that I was home for lunch to watch the full hour show. Captain Stubing, Gopher, Isaac, Doc, and Julie were having fun on a boat, and I could relate! It seemed that the full hour was devoted to trying to help people either fall in love or stay in love. By the end of the hour, love was surely found on that boat.

Peter found love on a boat–his boat. Shortly after calling Peter to leave his boat, Jesus used Peter's boat to give a speech to the people. When Jesus finished speaking he asked Peter to go out deeper so he would catch more fish. I wonder how Peter felt when Jesus started giving him fishing lessons? After all, Peter was the expert. I would have probably gotten upset that a carpenter was trying to give me fishing lessons! Peter, however, did not get upset. He knew there was something different about this carpenter from Nazareth. Peter did what Jesus asked him to do–he followed his directions. What happened next was miraculous! Peter caught such a large number of fish that the nets couldn't even hold the weight! The nets began to tear and break apart due to the amount of fish they caught. Even Peter knew this was a miracle because he knew that fish don't just jump into nets.

Sometimes I hear people say something to this effect, "If God would just show up and do a miracle, I would believe." I have to doubt the integrity of that statement. God does miracles all the time. He does many miracles that go unnoticed. Miracles like a baby being born, a golden sunset, a crisp evening, a hug, and a loving touch, or even a phone call. That day, God decided to do a miracle right in front of Peter's eyes. What was Peter's response? The Bible says that Peter, filled with amazement and awe, fell at Jesus' knees and said, "Go away from me, Lord; I am a sinful man!" Wow! That is such a peculiar response. Peter's response gives us insight into the man Peter knew he was. Peter on the outside was a strong and self-reliant fisherman, but on the inside he was sad. His sadness wasn't the kind of sadness you feel when you break up with your girlfriend; it wasn't the sadness you feel when you lose your job or you lose someone you love. Peter's sadness was the realization that he was not worthy of God's love. The light bulb came on for Peter. The windmill started working! God did a miracle right in front of his eyes, on his boat, and Peter knew he was in the presence of the living God.

Peter, realizing he was in the presence of someone greater than he, admitted his need for God and his shame of being in his presence. Peter was ashamed of who he was. He was ashamed that he had neglected God for some boats and some fish. At that moment, we get a glimpse of Peter's heart, a heart of humility. It takes humility to admit that you are a sinner, that you need God's forgiveness. Peter made an important admission, "I am a sinner, Lord, and I don't deserve your love." Peter admitted who he really was – a sinner, someone who had made mistakes and had regrets, someone who was trying to run his life and a business without inviting Jesus into his boat. That day, Peter decided to take step 1. He admitted he had a problem – sin – and that his problem was bigger than he was able to solve. He was now ready to take step 2. He was ready to believe.

A Door Knob

The point of step number 2 is to place your faith in a power greater than you and believe that your greater power can help you overcome your problem. I shouldn't have to say this, but be very careful about whom you choose as your higher power.

Once, while in an AA meeting, I heard a man say that he had finally found his higher power. He pointed at the door and told everyone, with excitement, that his higher power was the doorknob. He had looked at that doorknob every day, and for some reason he saw strength in the doorknob. I'm not questioning the sincerity of that man, but I would suggest that placing your faith in a doorknob is rather foolish. What can a doorknob do for you? Many people place their faith in things that are not powerful at all. Maybe they don't place their faith in doorknobs, but they do place their faith in other things like money, jobs, careers, and people. I knew a guy once that believed his 401k would be there to solve his problems once he retired, then the stock market crashed. I knew another person who believed that his health would never fail, and then he got diagnosed with cancer. Another person decided to place his faith in his friends, only to see them depart and never come back. There has to come a point when a person stops believing in things that won't last and start believing in something that will always last. Hope comes from believing in something better and bigger than you. If that "something" is anything other than God, you will be disappointed.

The God of the Bible

For years and years, people have placed their faith in the God of the Bible. Long before you or I were born, people with problems found the solution in the pages of the Holy Scriptures. Sadly, for most people, the God of the Bible is the last person they seek. There's a story of a man who fell off a cliff and miraculously grabbed a branch on the way down. As he was hanging on to the branch, he heard a voice saying, "My son, let go and I will catch you." "Who are you?" the man asked. "I am God, let go, and I will catch you." The man thought for a moment and then asked, "Is there anyone else up there?" Even though God was there to catch him, he was still looking for someone or something better. Why is it that God is the last person we trust to help?

The Bible is the story of God solving one problem after another culminating with the biggest problem of all, sin and death, which he solved on the cross. This is why Jesus said, *"What is impossible with man is possible with God"* (Luke 18:27). What was impossible for me to do on my own, heal and save myself, God did for me. What was impossible for Peter to do on his own, bring meaning and purpose into his life, God did for him. Will you give God a try?

God is Knocking at Your Door

You may not receive a phone call that will change your life, but you will hear a knock on your door. Jesus is knocking at your door. Will you answer? Peter was on his boat thinking about how bad of a person he was. "I don't deserve to be loved by anyone, especially God." Yet it was God in the flesh that was on his boat with him, and he was knocking on the door of Peter's heart. How do you know when Jesus is knocking on your door? You sense that your life is about to change. That is when you open the door to a power greater than yourself to come into your life and be the God of your problems and your life.

As you read the story of Peter's first encounter with Jesus, nowhere in that story do we read that Jesus kicked Peter off the boat. Nowhere do we read that Jesus got angry with Peter for asking questions. In fact, Jesus turned to Peter and said, "Peter, from now on you will be working for me; you will be fishing for people." In other words, "Peter, maybe other rabbis passed you up, but I'm not just any other rabbi, I am God and I am here to tell you that there is a bright future for you if you will just let me into your life."

That's the question. Will you let God be God in your life? Or will you try and overcome your problem on your own? Peter did eventually come to the realization of who Jesus was. Sometimes people think they have to have God all figured out before they trust him. That is not true. Peter took one step of faith and God revealed the next, then the next, and so on.

It was during a conversation Jesus was having with his disciples when Peter's windmill really started turning! Jesus was asking them who the people thought he was. Some said that they thought Jesus was a prophet, others said he was a good teacher, and still others said that he was a healer; but Peter, with confidence, said to Jesus, "You are the Christ, the living God" (Matthew 16:16). Everyone, at some point, has to make a decision regarding Jesus. Is he God, or is he just a good teacher, or a prophet, or a talented and gifted miracle worker? How did Peter get to such a place of confession? For Peter, it was a process. For me, it was a process. The key, however, in coming to an understanding of God, is curiosity. Curiosity may have killed the cat, but it gave life to Peter and to me. Peter was curious about his life and about God, curious enough to take a step of faith. I was curious about my life and about God. Even though I didn't know who he was, I kept the door opened, I prayed a prayer. That's why Jesus says, "Ask and it will be given to you; seek and you will find; knock and the door will be opened to you." (Matthew 7:7)

Sometimes It Takes A Miracle

Before my father passed away, I had the incredible privilege of seeing a miracle. As I mentioned, my dad suffered from diabetes. Because of diabetes, he had to have his leg amputated to just below his knee. As if that wasn't difficult enough, the infection came back, and the doctor, in an effort to save my father's life, ordered that his leg be amputated above the knee. This would have caused my father to lose the ability to have a prosthetic leg. My father was a man of deep faith. As we gathered around his bed before his impending surgery, he asked that we pray for God to heal his leg. He looked at me and said, "Son, I believe God can heal my leg." "Dad, I believe God can heal your leg too," I said. While in prayer, his leg moved. My father opened his eyes and asked, "Who touched my leg?" Someone touched my leg." With that, I responded, "I didn't touch your leg dad, but I prayed that God would touch your leg." After our prayer concluded, the nurse wheeled my father down to surgery. Around fifteen minutes later the doctor, dressed in his street clothes, came out and spoke to the family. He said these words, "I don't know how to explain this, but your dad's leg is totally healed. We do not need to amputate any more of his leg." I couldn't believe what I was hearing! Even though we prayed, I didn't think anything would change. Isn't that sad? I had just prayed to the God who created the universe, who spoke the world into existence; the same God who delivered so much fish into Peter's net that it broke. Yet I didn't truly believe he would help. But he did! God came through! My father's leg was healed! We experienced a miracle together; a miracle that not only changed my life, but also changed the lives of all involved, including the doctor, his staff, and the entire hospital. To this day, my father is known as the "miracle man" at that hospital.

I tell that story for two reasons: (1) To honor God and show that He is the One who can do miracles; (2) To show you that believing makes a difference! Healing Step 1 is to: Admit that you have a problem and need help solving it. Peter did this, I did this, and I hope you have done this too. Step 2 is to: Believe that God can solve your problem.

Healing Step 2: **Believe** that God can solve my problem and give me the help I need.

You've probably heard the saying that doing the same thing over and over again expecting a different result is the definition of insanity. For me, insanity was putting my faith in alcohol, drugs, music, and women, and expecting a better result. Those things, although at first were helpful in dealing with my problems, they wore out. The same thing happened with my willpower; my willpower wore out too. My dad, later in life, came to that same place, realizing that his willpower could only get him so far. He needed a miracle! The only thing that doesn't wear out is God's power, and He is sitting there in your boat just waiting for you to believe and ask for help.

Peter believed because he was curious enough to keep the door open. The worst thing anyone can do is shut the door to faith. What if God is real? What if he still does miracles? Wouldn't you want to know? Wouldn't you want him to do a miracle in your life? Are you tired of your problems? Are you worn out thinking about how to solve your problem? Jesus is saying this to you, *"Come to me all of you who are tired and worn out and I will give you rest"* (Matthew 11:48). Jesus wants you to come to him.

I encourage you to give God a chance. Maybe you've had bad experiences with God or with church. Maybe you've thought for the longest time God is mad at you. I know how you feel. I would suggest something to you right now – pray the prayer I prayed. *"God if you're real, please show me."* Maybe he is showing you. Maybe he will do something to show that he is God. Maybe he is in your boat with you and all you have to do is believe, ask that he open your eyes! Maybe you are reading this book, and you want God to do the same thing he did for Peter, show you who he really is. You want him to solve your problem. Maybe you need him to do a miracle like he did for my dad. What's the harm in asking? Jesus wants you to ask. He said that we do not have because we do not ask. He also said that if we knock, the door would be opened. The key is to first admit you have a problem and then believe that God can solve that problem. Are you willing to do this?

I will offer you two opportunities. First, I will give those of you who are ready the opportunity to place your belief in Jesus Christ, like Peter did. If this is something you want to do, then I want you to say these words out loud....

"Lord Jesus, I believe in you. I believe you are the living God. I believe that you came to live a perfect life, then die on the cross for my sins, because you love me. Thank you for dying on the cross for me, and I ask you to forgive all my sins. I place my faith in you now, and I give you my problem (name your problem if you know what it is). I believe that you are alive, and you are coming again to take me to be with you. Like Peter, I believe that you are the Christ, the Son of the living God. Please come into my life and help me. Amen."

If you prayed that prayer and meant it, then the Bible says that you are a new creation. You may not feel new, but according to God's Word you are. It is important now to continue to grow in your faith. I will help you with this through the rest of the book. I encourage you to give God your problems, to pray every day, and to ask for what you need. If things don't happen as fast as you think they should, don't give up! Remember, your miracle is just around the corner. The good news is that now you are not tackling your problems alone! Jesus is in the boat with you.

Maybe you're not ready to place your faith in Jesus Christ yet, but you are curious. You want to give God a chance to reveal himself to you first. If this is what you want, then I encourage you to say these words out loud....

"God, if you're real, please show me. I want to believe that you can help me, but I need to know for sure. I want you to reveal yourself to me in a real way. Help my eyes to be open to see your revelation. I want you to speak to me like you did Peter. Help me Lord to believe."

Step 3: Commit

"Nothing shapes your life more than the commitments you choose to make"–Rick Warren

 chicken and a pig were walking by a church where a gala charity event was taking place. Getting caught up in the spirit, the pig suggested to the chicken that they each make a contribution. "Great idea!" the chicken cried. "Let's offer them ham and eggs." "Not so fast," said the pig. "For you, that's a contribution. For me, it's total commitment!" Commitment is step number 3. Belief will get you in the door; commitment keeps you there. Commitment is a decision, a decision to go all in.

My wife Deborah and I have been married for 24 years. When we got married, we stood in front of people and in front of God and made a commitment, a commitment to stay together until "death do us part." We both have taken this commitment seriously. There have been times, especially early on, where walking out seemed like the only option, but we remembered the commitment we made to each other and stayed. We remembered how God had gotten us through previous rough patches, and we knew he would get us through our present rough patch if we remained faithful. Commitment is not based on a feeling; commitment is based on action. Some days I don't feel as much love towards my wife, but this does not mean that my commitment has changed. It only means that my feelings have changed. Feelings change all the time, but commitment never changes. Today it seems like commitment has taken a back seat to feelings. It has become an old-fashioned word that has lost its meaning and purpose. People don't take commitments seriously. I saw a billboard the other day advertising quick, easy divorce. It is amazing what commitment has become. Marriage is a relationship of commitment; so is our relationship with God.

Commitment to healing is a decision. It is a concerted effort on the patient's part to trust God's prescription for health rather than his own. I do not know what is best for me, only God knows. Therefore, it is best I trust his medicine over my own. When I would go to the doctor I would disregard his prescriptions, believing that he was just trying to sell me his latest pill. This is how I used to treat Jesus. I would ask for help, but then not trust his medicine. If someone truly wants to be healed, he must trust in his higher power. This is the subject matter of this chapter: Commitment. In this Chapter, we will speak of three areas of commitment: (1) Commitment to Christ (2) Commitment to The Word, and (3) Commitment to Each Other.

Commitment To Christ

By now, I hope you have come to a decision to trust in a higher power for your healing. My higher power is Jesus Christ. I hope that you will put your trust in him. I have tried all kinds of higher powers, and I can honestly say that Jesus is the most stable and trustworthy. Whether you trust in Jesus Christ or not, the point here is that you must realize that your problem is beyond your ability to solve. It can only be solved by a force or entity stronger and bigger than you. Once you admit that you have a problem and you are unable to solve it on your own, you believe that God is the one who can solve your problem, you are ready to take the next step.

Step 3: **Commit** my life and will over to the care of God.

"God" can mean many things to many people. Someone can say "Thank God" and I would not know which God they are referring to. When I speak of God, I am speaking of the God in The Bible. He is the God, according to the Bible, who created all things from nothing. He is the God of Abraham, Isaac, and Jacob. He made himself known to man and a nation called Israel. He then made himself known personally through his one and only Son, Jesus, The Christ. Jesus tells us, according to Scripture, that he is the full representation of God and has made God known to us (John 1:18). Therefore, if Jesus is the full representation of God, then he must know God. Furthermore, he must be God! You can read all throughout the New Testament about the miracles Jesus did while on this earth. Miracles that include healing sick people instantly, forgiving people's sins, walking on water, and raising dead people to life. This is what he did for me... he raised me from the dead. Someone may ask, "Did Jesus ever claim to be God?" The answer is yes. In many instances, Jesus claimed to be God. This is why the Jewish leaders wanted to kill him. He was, in their eyes, committing blasphemy. So, when I speak of God, I am speaking of God in the person of Jesus Christ.

It is important that you commit your life over to the care of God. The God you put your trust in should be capable of accomplishing miracles. He should be a God who can actually help you. I mentioned the man who put his trust in a doorknob. Seriously, I'm not kidding. The man's higher power was a doorknob! Now, maybe the doorknob gave him a sense of peace and care for a short time, but I can assure you that it did nothing to bring him everlasting care and comfort. Care and comfort come from someone who is tuned into your problems. This someone can only be someone who knows you like no one else knows you. This someone is the God of the Bible. In order to be healed, I must trust in something or someone greater than myself. For me, and I hope for you, this "someone" is Jesus Christ. This takes commitment: A commitment that never changes, even if my feelings change. This, after all, is God's commitment to you.

Here are three areas for which you should trust your higher power in regards to healing. You should trust him for: (1) Care (2) Comfort, and (3) Correction. Let's talk about each one.

God's Care

Did you hear of the man who was stuck in a tremendous flood? The floodwaters were overtaking him, and he could not swim. He mustered enough courage and strength to climb to the top of his roof where he prayed to God for help. At that moment, a boat came up to him. The boat captain looked at the man and said, "Jump in," to which the man answered, "I'm waiting for God to help me, so go on your way." As the water continued to rise, a helicopter flew above him, "grab on to the rope," the pilot said. "I'm waiting for God to help me, so go on your way," the man said. When the water was too high to navigate safely, he drowned. As he approached the throne of God in heaven, the man, in a humble voice asked, "Lord, I prayed that you would help me. Why didn't you help me?" To which God answered, "I sent a boat and a helicopter. What else did you want me to do?" This story illustrates how unaware and how unwilling we are in regards to God's help. When we pray, we either don't believe God can help, or we forget that we asked for help.

It is like the man who was on a cliff, lost his balance, and fell. On the way down, he was lucky enough to grab a hold of a tree limb. At that moment, he prayed, "God, help me!" That is when he heard a voice say, "My child, trust me to catch you. Jump!" "Who are you who speaks?" The man asked. "I am God," the voice answered." To which the man answered, "Is there anyone else who can help me?" The man prayed, but didn't trust. He prayed for God to help him, but would not submit to his plan; he didn't want to take the medicine. He didn't trust that God knew what was best.

As you realize, by reading chapter one, Bartimeaus was different than these men. He asked for help, and God healed him. Bart trusted God for the medicine because trust is an integral part of commitment. Without trust, commitment is meaningless. Jesus came to heal the sick, many of which were blind.

There's a story about a blind man who came to Jesus, and instead of being healed instantly, Jesus told him to go to the nearby pool and wash in it. The Bible tells us that this man went and washed and was healed. Can you imagine if God told you to do this? Would you go? Would you trust enough to leave and go? What's even more baffling is how Jesus chose to heal him. Before Jesus sent him to the pool, he took dirt from the ground, spit his saliva into the dirt, and rubbed it all over the man's eyes! That is weird! Can you imagine how this man would have felt? Yet, the blind man did not stop Jesus from applying the medicine; rather, because of his faith and trust, he went home healed. The point is this: <u>If you want to be healed by God, take the medicine!</u> God may send you to a "pool." He may send you to a doctor, a counselor, a friend. He may make your path to healing uncomfortable and messy. But the fact of the matter is, you don't know what medicine will work best for your healing. You're not the doctor. Therefore, you must commit to trust God for the medicine he gives you, no matter how messy or uncomfortable. Your problem can only be solved through supernatural deliverance. This is why trusting in God is the key to you being healed and your problem being solved.

Why do people reject God's medicine? This is partly due to the misunderstanding of how God works. Jesus tells us *"without faith it is impossible to please God"* (Hebrews 11:6). Therefore, if faith is the key to healing, I must let faith be activated. You already know that faith is the key to salvation, but it doesn't end there. Salvation is just the beginning. From the moment you place your faith in Jesus Christ as your Lord and Savior, God starts working in your life. The main ingredient he uses to accomplish his work is faith, along with his Spirit. If I am only willing to trust God for my eternal salvation, but not trust him for my daily problems, what does that say about my faith? What does that say about my commitment? The other reason people reject God's medicine is lack of commitment. It is always easier to do what I want to do rather than what God says to do. This is the plight of all humanity. Therefore, I fight the very one who wants to help me rather than trust him for the solution. He says jump, but instead I hold on. He says climb in, but instead I walk away. Your miracle may truly be just around the corner, but unless you walk to the corner, you won't receive it. God can't force you to walk. You have to be willing to walk.

The Man Who Couldn't Walk

In the Bible we read of a man who couldn't walk; he was paralyzed and unable to walk for thirty-five years. Every day he would go to the place where God would heal, a pool, and he would wait, hoping he would be healed. But for thirty-five years his healing never came. This man, though, kept showing up, and his tenacity paid off. One day while waiting, Jesus came to the pool of healing. He asked the man, "Why don't you jump into the pool to get healed?" His answer had a tone of helplessness, "Lord, every time the angel comes and moves the water, someone else jumps in before me. I can't move quick enough." Wouldn't it be amazing if at this moment Jesus picked the man up and threw him into the pool so that he could be healed? But Jesus did something even more amazing. He bypassed the pool and went directly to the source of the problem: "Stand up, pick up your mat, and walk!" Jesus proclaimed (John 5:8). At that moment, the Bible says that this man who was crippled and bedridden was instantly healed.

Put yourself in this man's position. For thirty-five years you were stuck to your mat. You had to rely on others to carry you to the place of healing. Then when you got there, you were never healed. Every day you went through the same routine, when finally Jesus shows up and says, "Get up and walk!" Would you walk? It always amazes me how God can bypass the "pool" so to speak, and go right to the heart of the problem. The "pool" is our medicine; it's what we think is best for us. But Jesus sees beyond the "pools" of our life to the root of the problem and says, "Get up and walk." The hard part about walking is that we have to do it. No one can walk for us. This man had to believe in his heart that the command, "Get up and walk," was what he truly needed to do. The pool wasn't working, so God had to bypass the pool.

How many years have you shown up, carrying your mat, hoping that the medicine in the pool would work? Are you going to keep doing the same thing? You know what they say about this type of behavior? It is called "insanity." And the definition of insanity is doing the same thing over and over expecting a different result. Isn't it about time to trust God to care for you? It might be scary, it might even get messy, but the end definitely supports the means because it leads to your ultimate desire – to be healed and for your problem to be solved.

God's Comfort

Commitment also involves trusting in God's comfort. I used to trust in the comfort of pills, but soon enough I realized the comfort only lasted a short time. Before long, I needed more "comfort". There's a reason they call the booze, "Southern Comfort". The problem is the name is deceiving. There is nothing comforting about getting drunk and waking up the next day worse off than the day before. Jesus came to give comfort and peace. This is what we need the most. He knows that this world is full of trouble, but he is bigger than the world, because he is the creator of the world. As a pastor, I have done my share of funerals. I have also shared in the grief of those who have lost loved ones. The best thing I can say in these situations is, "I'm sorry for your loss." There is nothing I can do, aside from praying, that will change their situation. We are mere humans and are subject to the pain of loss. However, there is a God who is not subject to these things, Jesus Christ our Savior. He not only understands our situation and cares, he can change the situation in an instant! This is the kind of God you should trust for your comfort.

God comforts us in times of trouble. When I am in trouble, I can talk to God, and I know he hears me. He can provide physical, emotional, and spiritual help. He may do this supernaturally, or he may choose to do this through another human being. There's a story of a woman who had just given birth to her baby. Her husband was out of work, and she was in serious need of help. The cupboard was bare and the fridge dry. She prayed to God that she would somehow be able to purchase milk for her hungry baby. That is when God sent a message, by his Spirit, to a man who seconds before was unaware of this woman's need. While driving down the street, he sensed God telling him to make some unplanned turns, which caused him to end up right in front of this woman's home. He knocked on the door, and said, "Mam, I'm sorry to bother you, but God told me that you needed this." He handed her enough money to go buy the milk she needed. These things happen all the time! The problem is that most people are clueless to the miracles God does on a daily basis. Someone who is committed to God not only believes God does miracles, he keeps an eye out for them!

The Thirsty Woman

While traveling from one city to the next, Jesus stopped for a drink of water at a well-known well in a foreign town. A thirsty woman showed up to draw water from the well. She came in the middle of the day just in time to meet Jesus. Jesus met this woman for a purpose. This woman was not only physically thirsty, more importantly she was spiritually thirsty. She was like a hot dry desert in the middle of the day. This is when Jesus spoke, "Will you give me a drink?" he asked the woman, to which she answered, "Sir, you are Jew, and I am a Samaritan woman. How is it that you ask me for a drink?" Jews were not supposed to associate with Samaritans, but Jesus didn't care. He knew that this woman was in need of spiritual care and comfort and was not going to let some human-made rule change his plan. This woman thought Jesus was interested in drinking the water from the well, but Jesus was more interested in offering this spiritually parched woman some living water. "Where is this living water?" the woman asked. From that question, Jesus took the opportunity to reveal things about her life that only God would know. "Go get your husband", Jesus requested. "I don't have a husband", the woman answered. "You are right, woman, that you don't have a husband; in fact you have had five, and the man you are living with currently isn't your husband" (John 4:17-18). Now, today, this would not be a big deal. Living together before marriage is a normal occurrence. But, back then, and rightly so, it was wrong. In fact it would have been a subject of shame. But that is not why Jesus brought this up. Jesus brought this up to show this woman her need for fulfillment. She was not happy. Anyone who gets married six times has deep internal problems that need to be solved. This revelation made by Jesus to this woman caused her to respond saying, "I know you must be a prophet." She then tried to deflect the conversation by speaking about religious topics. We often do this same thing. God reveals our need, and instead of admitting it, we deflect it. Jesus, however, was not going to let this unfilled, hurting woman get away without an opportunity to experience eternal healing. At a certain point in their conversation, Jesus revealed who he really is: "I am the Christ." On that confession, this woman believed. She went back to her town a changed woman. How do we know she was changed? She shared about Jesus with the entire town, and they all came to see Jesus, and many believed in him.

When God comes into our lives, we are changed from the inside out. Our emptiness is filled, therefore our spirit comes alive, and we experience spiritual healing. Our spiritual need is only found in Jesus Christ. We are spiritually parched, and we try to quench our thirst with physical water. What we truly need is spiritual water, water from a well that never runs dry. God's comfort comes when we believe in Jesus Christ as our Lord and Savior. It is at that moment that we receive living water; we receive the Spirit of God who fills our thirsty souls. This is when we can experience God's comfort. We can realize that we are never alone, that God is with us always because we have drunk from the well that never runs dry. God's Spirit is the one who quenches our spiritual thirst. His comfort is available to you today if you make a commitment to trust in God for your healing.

God's Correction

Do you remember ever hearing your parents say this: "This is going to hurt me more than it hurts you"? I didn't realize the truth of this statement until I had children of my own. It is hard to discipline my children because I love them so much; but is because I love them so much that I discipline them. I love my children so much that I want to protect them from harm, I want to help them grow up and make wise decisions, and I want to correct them before it's too late. In fact, a parent who does not discipline his or her child is questionable regarding their love for that child. This is how God loves his children: He disciplines them.

When I was in junior high, I had a P.E. teacher who was, in my opinion, over the top about discipline. He was like a sergeant in the army. Nowadays this teacher would have probably been disciplined because of how tough he was on the kids. We live in a "cupcake" world where kids have to be coddled. I am grateful for this fervent P.E. teacher. I learned a lot about the importance of preparation and commitment because of his disciplinarian approach. The difference between my P.E. teacher and God is that God disciplines those he loves. The P.E. teacher didn't love me; he was just trying to get me to do what he wanted me to do. God, on the other hand, disciplines me because he wants me to become the person he intends me to be. This is the wonderful blessing of being corrected by God. Since we are, through faith in Christ, God's children, God, our Father, will discipline us. Like that little child who, not realizing the danger, runs out into a busy street, God wants to protect us from the oncoming cars in our lives that could cause irreparable harm.

I made some bad decisions in my life. The effects of alcohol and drugs made my bad decisions even worse! One night, while in Hawaii, I inhaled so many drugs that I almost died. I did not listen to the voices of correction in my life. I continued to harm myself and, in turn, harmed others. I regret these things. I wish I could live my adolescent and young adulthood over again, but I can't. The good news, however, is that I don't have to be enslaved to my past. Jesus Christ's death on the cross and resurrection from the dead has given me a new life. By his grace I can start over. My new life began the moment I placed my faith and trust in him. Now, when I try and do something I shouldn't, I experience the correction of my Father in heaven. He cares about me a lot. Jesus said that since God cares for the birds by providing food and shelter, how much more will he care for me. The difference is that birds aren't known to sin. They don't do things they shouldn't. A cat may catch them sometime, but it is not due to their direct rebellion against God's standard. I, on the other hand, can make a direct choice to disobey God and, therefore, suffer the consequences. But it's not like I didn't know that it was wrong. I know when I am sinning. I know when I am rebelling against God. Not only do I know because of knowing what the Bible says, I know also because I have his Spirit living in me, convicting me. But think about this. Is this a bad thing or a good thing? Isn't it better to know that God cares enough to correct me so as to keep me from suffering harm? Wouldn't it be worse if he didn't care, and He just let me continue to harm myself and others? I am glad that He cares enough to correct me, to tell me right from wrong. Discipline doesn't feel good at first, but in the long term its dividends pay off. I'm glad that he wants to comfort me with correction.

The man whom Jesus healed at the pool was crippled for thirty-five years. In an instant he was healed. Jesus is good at healing. Do you know what else Jesus is good at doing? Telling the truth. After healing this man, Jesus told him something that should have sent shivers up his newly-constructed spine. "Stop sinning, or something worse may happen to you" (John 5:14). That is what Jesus told this man. Theologically, this brings into the picture some very important issues. First, what did this man do to become an invalid? The fact that Jesus told this man to stop sinning suggests that it was sin that my have caused this sickness in the first place. Or, it could just be that this man, during his thirty-five years, was involved with sinful behavior. I'm not sure what he could do since he could not walk. Plus, back then, there was no internet or platforms as such that could cause a crippled man to sin. I tend to believe that this man's paralysis and sickness were directly due to sinful behavior. Now, think about that. Jesus loved this man so much that even though he may have caused his own disease, he still had the willingness to touch him and heal him. That says a lot about who Jesus is and how much he cares for mankind. The decisions I make have an impact on my future. I know people who experimented with heroine, who are now either HIV positive or have contracted hepatitis. These people are forgiven of their sins by their faith in Christ, but they still carry their sin with them due to the decisions they made decades earlier. It is important to realize that sin carries with it serious consequences. Even though I am forgiven in Christ, I am also marred by the decisions I made. This is why God's correction is so important. If I hear the voice of God correcting me, and submit to his command, I can be spared a lifetime of regret.

Rebelling against God and his standards sometimes cause irreparable harm. This is why God cares so much about correcting us. In fact, I believe that the greatest act of compassion is God's discipline. I thank God that I can count on him, as my Father, to correct me when I am off-track. And I can count on his grace to forgive me when I mess up. It is better to stay on the path with God than to wander off into destruction. God's correction is an aspect of God's healing because it keeps me on the path. And God's correction can also take something I have done in the past and correct it so that I am no longer enslaved to it anymore. This is the best correction of all!

Commitment to The Word

In his book, *The Principal of the Path*, Andy Stanley says, "Direction – Not Intention – Determines my Destination."[1] I may have good intentions, but unless I have good direction, I may end up at the wrong destination. This means I must make whatever is most important my compass. Your compass should be infallible. Your compass should point north. This is the Word of God, the Bible.

An old sailor repeatedly got lost at sea, so his friends gave him a compass and urged him to use it. The next time he went out to sea, he got lost again. The compass was on his boat, but he did not use it. His friends again rescued him and asked, "Why didn't you use the compass?" The sailor responded, "I wanted to go north, but as hard as I tried to make the needle aim in the direction I wanted it to go, it just kept on pointing southeast." He was so certain he knew which way was north that he tried to force the compass to show north when he was heading south. He tossed the compass aside as worthless, and he failed to benefit from the guidance it offered. Too many people are trying to force "north" rather than trust north.

Jesus encourages us, in Matthew chapter 7, to build our house on the solid rock. He shares two examples, one example of what happens to a house that is built on the rock, another example of what happens to a house that is built on sand. The house that is built on sand is washed away by the storms of life, but the house on the rock lasts forever. Unless we are building our house, our life, on the solid rock of God's Word, we will be washed away.

I know that some who are reading this will give every kind of excuse as to why the Bible should not be trusted. I want to ask you, though, have you read it? Most of the people who have problems with the Bible have never even read it. How can someone make such an illiterate decision? Maybe you have read the Bible, and you can make an honest evaluation that it has not helped you. That I can accept. However, I will still challenge you as to whether you have applied what the Bible says to your life. For instance, the Bible says a lot about marriage. But I can honestly say that most of the couples I counsel, even though they have knowledge of what the Bible says about marriage, have not applied what it says to their own marriage. It's not enough to know what the Bible says. In order to have good direction, you must apply the message of the Bible to your life.

The Bible has a lot to say about healing. I have already shared stories about Bartimaeus and Paul. I have also shared stories of Peter and how God took him from an unknown fisherman to a well-known fisher of men. I want to now share a story about a woman who ran out of hope. She had a disease that caused her to bleed for twelve years! No matter what she did or whom she saw, nothing or no one could help. The Bible tells us that even though she spent all the money she had to get better, she just kept getting worse. She ran out of money and hope. One day she happened to find herself in a crowd of people. Jesus was in that crowd. She mustered up enough energy to push through the crowd towards Jesus. She came up behind him, reached out, and touched his cloak. That's when her bleeding immediately stopped! (Luke 8:44). This lady had no hope. She had no money. What she did have was commitment! She was committed to touching Jesus! Commitment can be the very decision that will heal you immediately.

I am a huge baseball fan. My favorite team is the Angels. Even though the Angels have the best player in baseball, Mike Trout, they haven't made it past the first round of the playoffs. In contrast, the Kansas City Royals have made it to the World Series two years in a row and won the World Series in 2015. They do not have the best baseball player, but what they do have is commitment. They are committed to the fundamentals of baseball – moving the base runner over, having productive at bats, pitching backwards and ahead of the batter. These fundamentals are what push a team full of nobody's to becoming a team of champions. The fundamentals for spiritual life, for Christian living, are found in the Bible, the Word of God. Commit yourself to these things, and you will experience healing and hope.

A Commitment to Each Other

On May 11, 1935, Bill W., the founder of Alcoholics Anonymous, encountered a threat to his newfound sobriety. During a business trip to Ohio, he found himself standing in the lobby of a hotel, craving a drink. With growing anxiety, he contemplated his options. Bill narrowed his choices to two: order a cocktail in the hotel bar, or call another recovering alcoholic and ask for help in staying sober. Bill knew that this choice came with high stakes. As an alcoholic who had nearly drunk himself to death, he'd endured four hospital stays for "detox". During his last visit, he'd hit bottom and cried out for divine mercy: "If there be a God, let him show himself." At that moment, Bill felt a white light blaze through his hospital room. He was seized with "an ecstasy beyond description" and concluded that he was free from any need for alcohol. But there was no divine blaze in the lobby of the Mayflower Hotel in Akron—only the dim lights of the bar and the lure of a drink.

Pacing through the lobby, Bill passed the bar and found a church directory. Within minutes, he was on the phone with a local minister. A series of calls put him in touch with an alcoholic surgeon named Dr. Bob. Bill arranged to visit the doctor at home.

Dr. Bob initially agreed to see Bill for only 15 minutes, but their meeting lasted for hours. Bill simply told of his drinking history, and Bob identified with it immediately. Bill thanked Bob for hearing him out—for his fellowship. "I know now that I'm not going to take another drink," Bill said, "and I'm grateful to you."

The key to sobriety for Bill was found in another person, his friend Dr. Bob. For Bill W., it was a life or death situation. He would either reach out to someone for help or take a drink and die. It is the same for those who are on the path to healing. It is either reach out or die. I know this may sound a bit melodramatic, but the fact of the matter is that for those who are serious about healing and recovering from years of abuse, commitment to accountability is of upmost importance. One cannot stay committed without the assistance of another person or a group of people who are headed in the same direction. This is the power we find in the Church. Although the Church has received bad press lately, the truth is that without other people who are heading in the same direction, we would lose our direction. We need each other. Paul Simon sang the song, "I am a rock–I am an island." People who think this way lead an empty, sorrowful life. No man is an island; all people are connected. Therefore, it is imperative to find people who are heading in the same direction you want to go. Those are the people who can help you stay committed on the path to healing.

Notice that I am very specific about who you should be associating with in regards to accountability. The people you associate with to help you stay committed must be people who are on the same path as you. Let's say you're on a hike and you come to a fork in the road. Which one do you take? The answer to this question depends on whom you are hiking with. Those who are serious about healing, will take the high road; those who are not serious, will take the low road and take you down with them. You have heard the saying "you become like who you hang out with." This is a true statement. One must realize that in order to reach the goal, one must be travelling with companions who are heading for the same goal. Healing steps cannot be walked alone. You must walk with healing partners, those who are willing to take the steps and willing to hold you accountable to taking them too. Don't try and heal alone. If you do, you will fall short of your goal. Find others who will heal with you. Commit to others who will in turn commit to you.

A Decision Has To Be Made

Back in 1963, John F. Kennedy announced publicly, "We're going to put a man on the moon by the end of the decade." That was the decision. Had all the problems been solved when he made that decision? No. Often times, we're afraid to make a commitment because we don't know what lies ahead. When I made a commitment to my wife and said, "I do", did I know that we were going to have 3 children, be called into full- time pastorate ministry to serve Jesus Christ in his Church? NO! When you make a commitment to something, you often times will not have all the answers.

Some people don't want to make commitments before they know all the answers. That never happens. You'll never know all the answers, and you'll never have all the problems solved. People who think this way are confusing the decision-making phase with the problem-solving phase. Successful leaders, business owners, entrepreneurs, millionaires, and billionaires – they all know one thing. They know to never, never confuse decision-making with problem-solving. The decision has to be made first, then the problem-solving can begin. The same thing happens with making a decision to commit your life to Christ – you need to make the decision to follow Him, then the problem solving can begin. The difference is that this time Jesus will be solving your problems. It's much better that way!

The prophet Isaiah made a decision without knowing all the details. While in a vision, he saw God seated on his throne in all his glory and majesty. It was an amazing experience for this young prophet. During this vision, he heard God ask for someone to step up and serve, "Whom will I send?" God asked. Isaiah answered, "Here am I, Lord, send me." When Isaiah raised his hand, did he know the assignment God had for him? No. He only knew that everything else paled in comparison to having an encounter with the living God. The irony is that Isaiah was sent to speak to a people who would not listen. Isaiah was assigned a job he could not do. In other words, Isaiah was a failure. Or was he? Is serving and living for God a failure? How can someone who serves the one who made him be a failure? We can't see all the things God can see. Therefore, we must trust God even when we can't see clearly the results of our labor. We may not have all the answers, but we can commit to the one who is the answer: Jesus Christ!

No Turning Back

One of the songs we used to sing to our children is the well-known hymn, "I have decided to follow Jesus." The lyrics simply say, "I have decided to follow Jesus, I have decided to follow Jesus, I have decided to follow Jesus. No turning back, no turning back." Commitment is a decision – a decision to follow no matter what. It is a decision to trust God for your healing no matter what he prescribes. This is the key to peace – it is the key to sobriety.

When Julius Caesar landed on the shores of Britain with his Roman legions, he took a bold and decisive step to ensure the success of his military venture. Ordering his men to march to the edge of the Cliffs of Dover, he commanded them to look down at the water below. To their amazement, they saw every ship in which they had crossed the channel engulfed in flames. Caesar had deliberately cut off any possibility of retreat. Now that his soldiers were unable to return to the continent, there was nothing left for them to do but to advance and conquer! And that is exactly what they did.

What are some ships that need to be burned? What is keeping you from making a commitment to following Christ? Those things that may seem good can be the very things hindering your healing. Maybe you need to burn some thoughts or feelings that are getting in the way of trusting God. Maybe you need to burn some experiences with church that have tainted your idea of what the church is and why it exists. You may need to burn some bad habits and get some new ones to replace them. Maybe you have been drinking from the wrong well, and it is time to start drinking living water. Whatever the case, remember that the A, B, C's of healing involves steps. You cannot get to the last step until you take the next one. <u>The next step is to commit your life to Jesus Christ so that he can care for you and heal you</u>. He is the one who can solve your problems. He is your healer.

Have you admitted that you are powerless over your problems and you can't solve them on your own? Do you believe that God can solve your problems and heal you?

If so, then you are ready to commit your life and will over to the care of God. I encourage you to pray this prayer:

"God, I offer myself to you to build with me and to do with me as you will. Relieve me of the bondage of self, that I may better do your will. Take away my difficulties, that victory over them may bear witness

*to those I would help of your power, your love, and your way of life.
May I do your will always."*

Step 4: *Discuss*

"The aim of discussion should not be victory, but progress" –
Joseph Joubert

"Confess your sins to one another so that you may be healed"
– James 5:16

On October 14, 1987, Jessica McClure, an eighteen-month-old baby from Midland, Texas, fell into a well. Over four hundred people took part in her fifty-eight hour rescue attempt, which was spurred on by her cries of anguish that could be clearly heard at ground level through a pipe. The rescuers decided that the rescue must have two phases: Phase one was to simply get someone down there, next to her, as soon as possible; phase two was actually extracting her from the well. Phase one was driven by the knowledge that people tend to do and think strange things when they are trapped alone in a dark scary place for long periods of time with no one to talk to. They get disoriented, and their fears get blown out of proportion. Their minds play tricks on them. Sometimes they start doing self-destructive things. Sometimes they just give up. The rescuers knew that if they didn't get someone down there with her soon, there would be no hope. Thank God that Jessica made it out safely. Somebody heard her cry! For many of us being heard is difficult either because no one listens or we don't talk. We feel like Jessica, stuck in a dark well, a dark scary place, where no one, it seems, cares or comes to our rescue. We do and think strange things, destructive things. This chapter will hopefully help you understand and implement the healthy habit of communicating through discussion.

Step 4: **Discuss** my problems with God and with other people

Dictionary.com defines the term *discuss* this way: <u>To talk over or write about</u>. One of the ways I discussed my feelings as a youngster was to write songs. The first song I ever wrote was for my fourth grade teacher. I wanted to tell her how much I appreciated her, and the best way I thought to do this was to write a song. Back then, we could not pull out a phone and record the song. I had to write the entire song out on music paper, and present it to her. The second song I wrote was ten years later when my high school friend passed away from a freak football injury. He injured his knee while playing the game and was taken to the hospital for knee surgery. While being operated on, he had a rare reaction to the anesthesia, which killed him. I was devastated. He was my best friend. Since talking was not something I would normally do, I decided to write down my feelings in a song and presented it to the family. Songwriting became my avenue of discussion.

Although writing songs is something I loved to do, it was not the most effective way to communicate. Writing a song could take up to weeks, sometimes months. Therefore, the entire time while I was writing, my feelings were being bottled up only to explode at inappropriate times. Whenever I would feel criticized, attacked, or treated badly, because I did not have a healthy habit of discussion, I would explode in anger. Being shy, I would not naturally speak to people. More than being shy, however, was my fear of opening up to people. I did not feel safe when speaking about my feelings. My parents were not good communicators either. Maybe they were as afraid of feelings as I was. All I know is that anytime I would want to speak about my feelings, I was shut down. I was not allowed to cry or be angry. Therefore, I bottled up my feelings and drank the feelings away. This, obviously, is not the way to be healed.

The Suitcase

We all have a suitcase we carry through life. Our suitcase has things we need but also things that we don't need, things that are weighing us down. For some, the suitcase has more of the latter than the former. Things like fear, discouragement, hurt, pain, broken dreams, fill our suitcase; and the heavier our suitcase, the bigger our problems. The key to peace and contentment is found in the ability to empty your suitcase of things that don't belong, and fill it with things that do belong. This can happen if you develop the habit of discussing your problems with God and with other people. We learn from discussions. When we discuss our problems we not only hear others speak, we also hear ourselves speak, which is extremely healing. My suitcase was filled with pain, anger, and unresolved feelings. My suitcase was so heavy that I could not carry it alone. Sadly, I felt like no one would help me carry it, so I just tried my best, but failed miserably. I felt like Jessica, trapped in a dark deep well where nobody could hear me. I was lonely and afraid.

The Power of Prayer

The importance of discussion rests in the fact that without it, people will die. We, as humans, are made to talk. We are made to talk first to God, and then to other people. We talk to God through what is called prayer. Prayer is simply talking to and listening to God. Although many people think prayer is difficult, it is not. Prayer is the easiest form of communication we have. I can pray anytime, anywhere, whenever. God never sleeps, so I don't have to wait until a certain time or place to talk. I can talk to God in the middle of the day or the depths of the night. There are many times when I will wake up in the middle of the night with fear or anxiety on my heart. It is then when I should speak to God. I should honestly communicate my feelings, fears, and anxieties, because the Bible says that I should *"cast my anxiety on him, because he cares for me"* (1 Peter 5:7). When you have a personal relationship with God through his Son, Jesus Christ, you have access to the most powerful force in the universe. God can move mountains, heal the sick, and raise the dead. Prayer is a lifeline that many people don't use. I encourage you to develop a healthy prayer life so that you can discuss your problems with God and watch for the results.

In this chapter I will speak of three topics of discussion. (1) Discuss your problems; (2) Discuss your sins; (3) Discuss your hope. I will speak of these three things in the context of prayer, but also in the realm of the material world by learning how to discuss your problems with another human being.

It is important to realize that the first thing God did in revealing himself to us was to speak to us through His Word. His Word, the Bible, is God's message to us. It is the ultimate form of prayer, because it is praying in his Spirit. But, our God isn't a distant God. God knew that the best way to communicate with us was to become like us, so he sent his Son into the world to live among us and talk to us. The message of Jesus is found in the Bible, and the Bible tells us that Jesus is the exact representation of God (Hebrews 1:3). You can find out what he said by opening up the pages of Scripture.

If your dog was sick and would not take his medicine, what would be the most effective way of communicating to him the importance of taking his medicine? You would become a dog! We, as humans, are sick. We are infected with a disease that is killing us. God, in his ultimate wisdom, became one of us, to tell us to take our medicine – to find hope and forgiveness in our Lord, Jesus Christ. He is the one who saves us and heals us of our spiritual sickness. He is also the one who is seated at the right hand of the Father praying on your behalf. Did you know Jesus is praying for you? Since he is praying for you, why not talk directly to him through prayer? But also, find other human beings, people like you, with whom you can discuss your problems.

Discussing Your Problems

If you turn to the pages of Psalms in the Bible, you will find some incredible discussions going on between the psalmist (the person who wrote the psalm) and God. Psalms are like songs. We don't really know the melody of these psalms, but we are well acquainted with the lyrics – lyrics about pain, anger, frustration, loneliness, and depression. The psalmist was able to get through his day and his life by discussing his problems with God and writing them down. Discussing your problems with God is a key to experiencing your healing. But the Bible also gives us insight into the importance of discussing our problems with other people.

The Bible is full of documented incidents of people talking to God and to others about their problems. One of the most notable is in the Old Testament, found in the Book of Job. Job was a man who lived in a time when people were either for God or against God, much like the time we live today. The story of Job starts out by explaining that he was a very wealthy man with many children. He was blessed with many blessings and he was a man who sought after God. The story takes a dynamic shift when the scene changes to heaven. The scene change opens with God speaking to a very suspicious character. The character God is speaking to is the Devil, also known as Satan. God asks Satan a question regarding Job. He asks, "Have you noticed my servant Job, how much time he thinks about me, how many things he does for me? He is a faithful person." Satan responds by saying, "Well, God, that's because you bless him. I bet if you stopped blessing him, he would stop blessing you and start cursing you." God takes the bet, but with a condition … that Satan is not to touch Job himself. So Satan hurries to earth, wasting no time, he causes problem after problem in Job's life.

First, he causes some of his children to be murdered by foreigners, next he causes his house and property to be burned up in a fire, then he kills his servants in a massacre; and finally, his children who didn't die in the murderous attack, die when their house falls on top of them in a wind storm. Job, who had everything, now had nothing. He sat and cried, as he grieved of his loss, but never once blamed God. Instead, he just accepted all these problems as God taking things away that were once give to him. Job, who didn't have any problems, now had many problems.

The next scene shifts back to heaven where Satan is again speaking to God. God acknowledges Job as a man who maintains integrity even in the midst of horrible circumstances. Satan wastes no time in blaming Job's persistent integrity on the fact that God held back and didn't allow the Devil to touch Job himself. Then God does something incredible. He gives Satan permission to do whatever he wants with Job as long as he doesn't kill him. Satan wastes no time attacking Job with a painful skin disease. As he sat there in terrible pain, his wife encouraged Job to lose his integrity by cursing God. Job's response is very telling about his character. He says to his wife, "How can you talk like that? Are we to just expect good things from God and not trouble?" All the while, no matter what the problem, Job trusted and believed God.

Now, before you start comparing yourself to Job, let's consider some things about this story. First, let's consider the fact that there are two distinct places mentioned in this account of Job's life – heaven and earth. Job is on earth; God is in heaven. Heaven and hell are real places. Second, consider that there are two entities included in this story, God and Satan. The fact that they are conversing, tells us that they exist and they communicate. It is evident that things are going on in heaven that we cannot see or know. The only way we know of this conversation between God and Satan is because it is written in the Bible. However, most people live like there is only one dimension – earth. They rarely, if ever, think about heaven or eternity. The perspective we hold on earth will affect how we live and what we believe about problems on earth. According to the Book of Job, God and Satan speak. Also, according to this book, Satan must ask permission to annoy or touch one of God's servants. Job believed in God, therefore he was one of God's own. If you believe in God, through His Son, Jesus Christ, then you are one of God's own. This means that God's hand of protection is on you. But, what about ... when God allows trouble? What about when God allows problems to come into your life? Do you see those problems as God hurting you or helping you? Why did God allow problems into Job's life? Did God allow the problems to happen to hurt Job or to help him? I'm going to tell you the end of the story. This is a spoiler alert! The end of the Book of Job we find out that God blessed Job with even more blessings than he had in the beginning. The Bible tells us that God gave Job his children back (well, not his old children, but new ones), his money back (much more than he ever had), and his joy back. But it was a long process. Why did God allow this to happen?

The Test

The thing about tests is that they can cause much stress. Just a few years ago I decided it was time to go back to college to obtain a Master's Degree. The first time I had to take a test, I freaked out! I am a perfectionist by nature, which means I do not like to make mistakes. Therefore, testing causes me much anxiety! Job was tested by God. God allowed things to happen in Job's life so that his faith would be tested. Most people don't like tests, but tests are how we grow. Some of your problems may be due to a test. There's a saying that goes, "God wants to turn your test into a testimony." God is allowing things into your life to see how much you trust him. I'm not saying that all your problems are tests, but understanding that God uses difficulties this way can help you see the reality of the situation. The reality is that God sometimes allows situations and circumstances into your life so you will grow in your faith. Faith is like a muscle and only grows when tested. It's not that God is trying to hurt you; he is actually trying to help you – help you grow.

Although tests are stressful, the more you take tests, the more comfortable you become. It is the same with our problems. When we can see our problems, not just as problems, but also as tests, we can become more and more comfortable if we give our problems to God and trust Him to help us get through it. God doesn't expect us to take the test alone. He desires us to ask for help. He desires that we talk about our problems so we can grow in faith rather than shrink in fear. Job was tested, and Job passed the test. How did he pass the test? He discussed his problems with his friends, and he trusted God to get him through it.

The Discussion

Job had a long discussion with his friends, thirty-six chapters to be exact! The discussion was not very fruitful. Job's friends did not show much mercy or compassion for their friend, Job. They blamed Job for what was happening. These are the kinds of friends nobody needs! Sadly, these are sometimes the friends we talk to during trials and tests. Friends like these tend to try and fix the problem rather than just listen. When discussing your problems with someone, it is important to discuss with people who have a sensitive ear, someone who will listen and not try to fix your problem, because they cannot fix it. Only God can fix it. Choose friends who can lend an ear, friends who will listen as you talk. Discussing your problems with someone does not necessarily promise an outcome, as much as it offers an outlet. Talking about your problems with someone takes it from internal to external. A fire hose is of no good unless the water comes out. Our mouth is of no good unless the words come out. This can be difficult for someone who is shy or introvert. However, it is so important that even if it is uncomfortable, you must do it. It is a life or death situation.

Even though Job did not have much success discussing his problems with his friends, at least he discussed them. At least he got it off his chest. I'm sure he felt at least somewhat better just sharing his struggles with another human being. Do you remember the movie Castaway? In this movie, Tom Hanks plays a castaway stuck on an island all alone. He was stranded on that island for many months. During his time on the island, he built shelter and caught food, but he was lonely. It was the loneliness that was hardest for him. One day he found a volleyball that washed up on shore. He drew a face on the ball and named it Wilson. Wilson saved his life! We realize how important Wilson was to this castaway when Wilson was washed away one day while the castaway was floating on his man-made raft. The castaway cried and cried when he realized Wilson was no longer around. This shows the importance of communication with another human being. Even though Wilson was just a ball, it still helped save the man's life because the castaway had an outlet to speak. Speaking helps solve your problem, and keeps you from digging a deeper hole.

Discussing Your Sins
(Confession)

Due to my Catholic upbringing, I am very familiar with the idea of "confession". It was important to confess to a priest on a regular basis so that I would be forgiven. I would enter the confessional, be it scared, and share my sins with another human being who was shielded from view by a dark curtain. Although this habit of confession is important for our well-being, this particular process is not the best way to handle confession. The Catholic Church has the right idea, but the wrong implementation. James 5:16 says, *"Confess your sins to one another, so that you may be healed."* Notice it says to confess your sins <u>to another person</u>. Confessing to another person is biblical. But the person to whom you confess should be out in the open, not behind a curtain. Notice it says, "confess your sins to *one another*." The *one anothers* are people who are the same in nature. When confessing you should speak with people who are like you, who have the same goal – walking a path of healing relying on God's power.

It is important to understand that forgiveness of sins comes from God, not from a person (1 John 1:9). Therefore, confession should be employed on a regular basis, but with people whom you trust. Trust is an important aspect regarding confession, and trust is earned. Confession involves admitting your mistakes, your struggles, and agreeing that these things are wrong. For instance, if I struggle with viewing pornography, and I sin by viewing it, I should first admit that this behavior is wrong. Second, I should confess this to God by agreeing it is wrong. Third, I should confess my sin to another person. Why is it important to confess to another person? One word: <u>Accountability</u>. Many people run from accountability, "I don't want anyone knowing what I'm doing or telling me that what I'm doing is wrong." Here's the deal: <u>I cannot get over my problems if I won't get over my pride</u>. The Bible tells me that God opposes people who are proud, but gives grace to the humble. Pride is what keeps God away; humility opens up the door to healing. In other words, if I am too prideful to admit that I am not perfect, if I am too arrogant to admit my mistakes to God and to another person, I will never heal.

Take the First Step

One of my greatest joys in life was seeing my children take their first step. When they were born, we lived in a very small condominium. There was no room to walk or run. But when we moved to a bigger house, my children started to walk and run! Seeing them take their first step was amazing, but hearing their first words was astounding! It is a wonderful blessing to be present when children are learning to talk. At first, their words sound like a foreign language, incomprehensible. It isn't long, though, that syllables begin to form together to make intelligible words. Then they grow up, and you wish they would stop talking! There is a difference, however, between forming words and talking. Anyone can form words. Talking, however, is much more advanced. As a child, I learned how to form words but I did not learn the art of talking.

My week in the hospital (rehab) was a learning experience. I learned that I am not as strong as I thought I was. I learned that I needed help. And I also learned that in order to get help, I needed to talk! Upon returning home from the hospital, I needed to start implementing the things I learned so that I would never end up there again. The most important thing, as far as I am concerned, was to implement the art of discussion – to talk things over. But who would help me? I needed help, and God sent the right man. This man became a major force in keeping me mentally stable and healthy. I did not know this man before I went into the hospital, but he became my best friend. He heard of my plight and called me the day after I returned home from rehab. He told me of a very important meeting I needed to attend and that I should go. He gave me his phone number and said these three very comforting words, "Call me anytime." I responded to him by asking, "What if I need to call you at 4 a.m., is that okay?" "Yes, any-time," he answered. He then said something that I had never heard before, "David, what you don't understand is that I get as much out of helping you as you get by being helped." Those words changed my view of why people help other people, and what should be the attitude of a helper. I took him up on his offer, and I started to learn how to talk again.

My first Twelve Step meeting was eye-opening, to say the least. There I was, with one hundred other men, who were very open about their feelings. The meeting started with some announcements, a prayer, and then a time of sharing. It was amazing to hear the stories these men were sharing. One man said that he used to live in a cardboard box under a freeway overpass. Another man told of a time when he thought he killed someone while driving drunk, but the person lived. The men shared their stories so honestly and openly. I had never seen or heard such a thing. Hearing these men speak so openly about their struggles gave me perspective: "I'm not alone." There is always someone who is worse off than me. But the only way I can know this is to hear it. As a friend of mine always says, "I have to show up and suit up." When I start to feel like Jessica–alone and afraid, I must suit up and show up to the discussion. Even if I don't speak, at least I can hear others speak of their problems. This helps me heal.

My friend told me that I should attend forty meetings in forty days. Since I had been through the ringer, and realized my stubborn tendencies, I decided to listen to him the same way I listened to the doctor in the hospital. I attended forty meetings in forty days. I attended morning meetings, noon meetings, and evening meetings. Sometimes I went to meetings twice a day. My first reaction to meet-ings was that I really didn't feel like I belonged there; they were different than me. However, not too long into the forty days, I realized that I did belong there; not only that, I was just like them! I began to find myself in their stories, and it wasn't long till I raised my hand to present my first "share".

You would think, being a performer, that speaking in public came easy for me. That is far from the truth! In fact, I am an incredibly shy person. When God asked me to start The Gate Church, I debated with him as to who would be the speaking pastor. I was sure it would not be me, because I was not adequate enough for the job. I felt more comfortable singing behind a piano; but sharing, especially sharing my feelings, was incredibly scary. It is interesting that for so many years, I would share my feelings through songs and not think twice, but for some reason, speaking my feelings felt, at the least, awkward, and at the most, terrifying.

I remember the first time I prayed in public. It was shortly after being hired at Saddleback Church. I remember telling God that he had permission to ask me to do anything, but "please don't ask me to pray in public!" I finished the last song, and it was as if God wrote in the sky, "pray"... so I did! My prayer was juvenile and simple, but after I prayed, the pastor in charge first complimented me on my singing, but then said, "I really loved your prayer." Hearing him say that opened up a door of confidence. From that moment on, I was less terrified to pray in public, and more interested in praying honest, sincere prayers so that others could sense the presence of God. Sharing my first "share" in that twelve step meeting was similar to praying in public for the first time. I stumbled through sharing about how broken I was, and how scared I was, and when I finished, they thanked me and moved on. There wasn't a pastor who spoke encouragement to me; there wasn't even anyone who encouraged me except a couple of people after the meeting. I knew, though, that sharing my feelings in public was the right thing to do. I started to feel safe. No one judged me; no one laughed or mocked me. They just listened, and I talked. Talking that day was kind of like letting some pressure out of the balloon. Every time I shared, a little more pressure escaped. It felt right. It was right. At forty-three years old, I was learning how to talk for the first time!

Having friends who listen is a wonderful gift. Knowing that I can be honest and open is tremendously healing. As I write this, I am reading of a man who, during a terrorist attack in San Bernardino, wrapped himself around a younger victim, and said, "I got you." He saved this person from dying. Being involved in a discussion group is like hearing the words, "Don't worry, I got you." I may not even know these people, but the fact that they know what I struggle with helps bring peace and healing to my life. I have learned that talking is essential to my well-being. It is essential to your well-being too. Find a place, a safe place, where you can be yourself, where you can take off your mask, and share your problems.

Discussing Your Hope

Flagstaff, Maine, is a town that no longer exists. The need for electric power to the rest of Main was so great that Central Main Power decided that it would have to open the dam and flood the city of Flagstaff in order to save the rest of Maine. Flagstaff was doomed. And ironically, the river that was about to flood this city was called, "The Dead River." Because of this, all improvements to the city stopped. Since the city was about to drown under water, why spend money and time fixing it? In 1949, the waters came and swallowed up this hopeless town. Flagstaff Lake is now the largest man-made lake in Maine. You can actually canoe over where people lived. When did the town of Flagstaff die? Was it when the waters came? No, this town died the moment it lost hope; the moment it heard the news of impending doom. When there's no hope in the future, there's no power in the present.

Hope is the key to your success! When I had sunk to my deepest depression, I found that I was losing hope. In fact, when visiting the psychiatrist the day before I ended up in rehab, she asked me, "where is your faith?" She had assumed I had lost my faith. I hadn't lost my faith. I have never lost my faith. What I lost was my hope, and hope is the fuel for my faith. Therefore, losing my hope caused me to want to lose my life. If I won't discuss my problems with another person, I will end up dying in a dark deep well. I will lose hope. It is that simple.

Hearing people speak of hope gives me perspective. When we had our twins, Austin and Ciera, we were overwhelmed! I remember my wife, Deborah, telling me that she had two dogs once and couldn't even take care of them! How could we take care of two kids at once? I remember I started to invite myself to my own pity parties. I started complaining about how hard my life had become. That was until I saw parents with triplets! Hearing other people speak of their problems and the hope they have, gives me proper perspective. I'm not alone, and my life isn't that bad. If I stay in the cave, in the dark, I will never know about the light of hope that lies right outside my door. I need to hear how others made it through, so that I can have hope too! But, I shouldn't just wait to hear from others. I must also share the hope I have. You may not see hope right now, but I promise you that one day you will. As soon as you start to see even a glimmer of hope, share it! Hope is the light that brightens my path!

Share The Road

 The night was dark driving home on the canyon road from a 12-step meeting. It was early on in my healing step journey, and I was feeling discouraged. I had been out of the hospital long enough to get back to my previous life, but not long enough to get my feet back on the ground. This new life was hard to get used to. As someone told me, "you are getting used to your new normal." I didn't like how this new normal felt! There were so many changes happening, that I doubted if I could make it through. I was talking to God in prayer on the way home, asking him to please reveal his plan to me. I felt alone and needed some encouragement. It was then that my headlights shined brightly on this sign: "Share the Road." The sign is intended to remind drivers to share the road with bicyclists, but to me it had an entire different meaning. God spoke to me through that sign. He said that he wanted me to share the road I was on with others. That sign helped give me perspective as to why I was going through what I was going through.

One of my favorite verses in the Bible is this: *"God comforts us in our troubles so we can comfort others with the same comfort we ourselves received from God"* (2 Corinthians 1:4). God showed me the sign to tell me that he wanted me to share the road, so that others will be encouraged and comforted. That is part of the reason I am writing this book. I want to share my road with you, so that you might find comfort and encouragement to stay on the path to healing. From that moment on, after I saw the sign, I had a new perspective. Even though I knew I had a long road ahead of me, I was ready to accept God's plan, so that He might be exalted through my trials.

The way I shared the road, at first, was through sharing at 12-step meetings. I would share my story in hopes that someone might find hope. This is the beauty of discussion. Discussing our problems with God and with others not only helps us, it also helps others. During this time, I would also share the road at church. I would share with my congregation the struggles I had and the pain I was experiencing. I remember the time I stood up in front of my congregation. The church was only two years old at the time. One Sunday morning I told them, "I have carried you for two years, now I need you to carry me. I need your help." This was a very humbling step to take, to stand in front of those who counted on me and ask them to help. Some people would just hold it in and not share, but I could not live like that any longer. I had to ask for help. What came out of that was so beautiful. The members of my church took it upon themselves to start a 24/7-prayer team. They stood in line to sign up to pray for me! After signing up, they gave me the list as encouragement. They told me that whenever I would wake up in the middle of the night I could look at the names of those who were praying for me during that exact time. It was so amazing to feel this kind of love from them.

Another time, while at a community prayer night, the pastor asked if anyone needed prayer to please come up and share. I remember sitting in my chair thinking, "I'm not going up there. I don't want to put myself in such a humiliating situation." Those thoughts were coming from the old me; the person who would wear masks hoping people wouldn't see the hurt that was inside me. I knew now that I could not let those thoughts dictate my actions any longer. I had worn a mask for too long. The mask was coming off! I went to the front, and with tears shared my need for prayer. You see, not only was I experiencing emotional pain, I was also experiencing physical pain. I had developed a stomach disease that would eventually lead to surgery. My problems were mounting, and I needed to share the road so I could heal. I went to the front and asked for prayer.

What happened next blew my mind. Not only did the entire congregation of around two hundred people pray for me, but also God spoke to someone in the congregation to come forward and help me. In the congregation that night was a doctor who specialized in my illness. He gave me his number and asked me to set up an appointment. He told me he would treat me for free a few times. I took him up on his offer. That doctor was instrumental in helping me get to another level in my healing. The only reason the doctor knew about my problem was because I talked about it with other people. What if I remained silent that night? I may have missed my healing. That is why it is so important to discuss your problems with other people. You never know who is in the audience.

There's a story of a cemetery that didn't bury the dead deep enough. When a flood hit, the dead bodies started coming out of their graves. That's what happens when we don't talk. We bury our feelings, our guilt, our resentment; but when life gets tough, as it most surely will, those feelings rear their ugly heads and come out of their graves. They cause deep problems in our lives and in the lives of the people we love the most. I encourage you to take this step. I encourage you to hang around people who are honest and sincere, people who will listen to you, and not try to fix you, because no one can fix you, except God. Discussing your problems is not the end; it is the means to the end. Sharing the road you are on is important, not only to your healing, but also to the healing of others. It has been said that God never wastes a hurt; that he wants to turn your mess into a message. He wants you to share the road, and trust him for the outcome.

If you are ready to take this step, I invite you to pray this prayer:

"Lord, I want to take this step of discussing my problems with you and with other people. Cause me to be honest, so that my suitcase can become lighter. I am tired of carrying around unresolved feelings and emotions that are weighing me down. Please remove my pride and fear, and cause me to take this step. I want to come out of the dark into the light. I ask that you lead me to people who will be sincere and honest with me, who will help me get things off my chest, so I can have perspective. I want to share the road, so that others can heal too."

Step 5: *Embrace*

"For to me, to live is Christ and to die is gain" – Philippians 1:21,
The Apostle Paul

In the fall, Linda, a young woman, was traveling alone up the rutted and rugged highway from Alberta to the Yukon. Linda didn't know that you don't travel to Whitehorse alone in a run-down Honda Civic, so she set off where only four-wheel drives normally venture. The first evening, she found a room in the mountains near a summit and asked for a 5 a.m. wakeup call so she could get an early start. She couldn't understand why the clerk looked surprised at that request, but as she awoke to early- morning fog shrouding the mountaintops, she understood. Not wanting to look foolish, she got up and went to breakfast. Two truckers invited Linda to join them, and since the place was so small, she felt obliged. "Where are you headed?" one of the truckers asked. "Whitehorse", she answered. "In that little Civic? No way! This pass is dangerous in weather like this." "Well, I'm determined to try", was Linda's gutsy, if not very informed, response. "Then I guess we're just going to have to hug you", the trucker suggested. Linda drew back. "There's no way I'm going to let you touch me!" "Not like THAT!" the truckers chuckled.

"We'll put one truck in front of you and one in the rear. In that way, we'll get you through the mountains." All that foggy morning, Linda followed the two red dots in front of her, and she had the reassurance of a big escort behind her, as they made their way safely through the mountains.

Sometimes we need to let God hug us, to reassure us of his love. We need to follow the big red dots of his Word to get us home safely. He embraces us as we embrace his will for our life. He keeps us safe and shows us the way home. Jesus tells us that if we seek God's kingdom first, everything else will fall into place (Matthew 6:33). God's kingdom is where God reigns, and he wants to reign in your heart. When you do this, the fog will lift, and you will see clearly his plan for your life. Embracing God's will for your life is the best hug you can ever get, because his plan for your life is incredible!

Step 5: **Embrace** God's Will for My Life

Before someone dies, hopefully they will draft a will. A will is something that directs the affairs and resources according to the will of the one who died. If someone does not have a will, then his or her hard-earned money will be doled out according to the will of someone else, not the owner. God's will is similar in that it is according to his desire that his will is doled out. In other words, his will is his demand, and he gives according to his purpose. He is the one who owns all resources; therefore, he wills it according to his purpose. This can either be good or bad according to how one views God. If someone views God as unloving, then they will see his will as a bad thing; but if someone views God as loving, then they will accept his will as good, no matter the circumstances. For, if God is a loving God, then he will give according to his love.

The Bible tells us that God is love; therefore, everything he does is based on love. His love is not a human love; his love is divine. In fact, his love is the basis for who he is. "God is love" (1 John 4:8). Notice it doesn't say that God is *about* love, *interested* in love, or even *loving*. It says that God **is** love. His very being is love. Everything he does is done in love, because he is the very essence of love. This means that when I accept God's will for my life, I accept his love into my life; the very creator of the universe is hugging me!

There are three aspects to God's will that I want you to embrace: (1) God's Will; (2) God's Word; (3) God's Work. Let's talk about each one.

Embracing God's Will

Let's say that I wanted to give you a gift, and I told you it was the best gift you would ever want to receive. You would probably question me because I don't know anything about you. How could I know it is the best gift you could ever receive if I don't know anything about you? This is the problem with humans ... we are finite and fallible. God, however, is infinite and infallible; he is love. He is omniscient and all-knowing. Therefore, he can give gifts that are especially made for the person receiving the gift.

When I was young, I believed in Santa Claus. I would always be amazed on Christmas, how amazing Santa was that he knew exactly what I wanted. I later learned that it was not Santa at all; it was my parents all along who gave the gifts. How did Santa know what I wanted? He didn't; but my parents knew, and the gifts were perfectly ordered for me because they loved me. If you have placed your faith in Christ, then God is your Father. He knows all about you and knows what is best for you. The problem with God's will sometimes is that the very thing we need may be the very thing we don't want.

The Rolling Stones wrote a song that says, "You can't always get what you want....but if you try sometime you find you get what you need."[1] What you want and what you need may be completely different. This is the challenge with embracing God's will for your life. God knows what you need, which often times causes a battle between your will and God's will. But if God owns everything, and he wants to give according to his desire and love, then fighting God's will for your life is like fighting against the very thing you need, which leads to regret and disappointment.

From the Beach Boys to Saddleback

As I mentioned earlier, touring with bands like Mike Love and the Beach Boys was exciting, but it was unfulfilling. Yet as unfulfilling as that may have been, even more unfulfilling was playing in local nightclubs. Back when I played in nightclubs, smoking cigars and cigarettes was allowed. I hated cigarette and cigar smoke! I would bring a fan and blow the smoke back into the audience's face. The smoke was extremely offensive and caused me to get sick. After placing my faith in Christ, I knew that the clubs were not where I should be. I needed to get out of the fog and into the light. Performing in clubs brought me to places where I had struggled and, therefore, caused me to want to leave them as quick as possible. But I knew that God had a plan. I remember praying, "Lord, if you want me to stay in the clubs I will, but I'd rather serve you full time."

It was December 1992. Deborah and I had been married for 6 months, when we arrived home from a trip to see her parents, to a phone message on my recorder. The phone message was from a friend of mine with whom I attended college. He left a message about a church in the Saddleback Valley that was looking for a musician who could do what I do – play piano and direct choirs. The church, I found out, was Saddleback Church, which at the time was one of the largest churches in America with 6,000 members. My wife, in her encouraging way, said, "You'll never get that job. That's a huge church!" Needless to say, I did not feel ready or equipped to take the job, but decided to send a resume anyway. I received a call to come and meet with the worship pastor, and a couple of weeks later I was hired! They hired me to be an assistant worship leader, someone who would lead worship through music on Wednesday nights and for the youth program, as well as play piano for the choir. Playing piano for the choir was something that didn't scare me, and playing music for the youth didn't either, since I had taught high school in the past. But leading worship for adults was another thing! I was so out of my comfort zone that I didn't know where to start. In fact, I didn't even know any Christian worship songs. I spent the first few months just sitting in a closet at Saddleback Church listening to worship songs and learning them.

I remember so clearly the first Wednesday night I led worship. I was so scared. I felt like a fish out of water. I remember praying this prayer that very first night: "Lord, I will play music for you, but please don't ask me to pray." I was in no way, ready to pray pub-licly! As I led worship that night, I was blessed. Hearing the people sing along with me was so encouraging. When I got to the end of my music set, there was a long pause. During the pause, I felt the urge to pray. So I prayed. I don't remember the specific prayer, but I do remember it being a prayer of gratitude for the sunshine and for the time we had together. It was not a long prayer, and to be honest, was rather sophomoric. After the night was over, the pastor in charge came up to me and said these words: "You did a great job tonight with the music, but I especially liked your prayer." It was as if God was giving me a big hug! I felt so encouraged.

The point of me telling you this is that embracing God's will always involves faith. Faith is being sure of what you hope for, and certain of what you do not see (Hebrews 11:1). Faith is uncomfortable, but without faith it is impossible to please God (Hebrews 11:6). It is impossible to please God without faith, because faith is what leads someone into the arms of God.

Many people operate on the basis of fear rather than faith. The night I led worship for the first time, I was scared. I did not want to do it. It was uncomfortable. But it was faith that caused me to do it even when I was scared. In fact, faith is the opposite of fear, because faith is moving forward in spite of fear. And to think that the first step of faith I took that night has led to over 20 years of serving the Lord in leading people into God's presence through worship. I shudder to think where I'd be if I didn't take that first step. But there are many people who, because of fear, because of doubt, miss out on God's will. The fog clouds their view of reality. Don't let that happen to you. Embrace God's will, because it is his will that will lead you to his embrace, which leads you to where God wants you to be, and ultimately to where you want to be.

Embrace God's Word

How do I find out God's will for my life? Wills are written out. When someone dies, they read the will to find out what is in it. God's will is written out – in the Bible. The Bible is the most read and most sold book in the history of the world. It has outlasted wars, mockery, persecution, and rallies to extinguish it. The Bible is the only book that has been written by 40 authors in different places at different times, yet has the same message. It's hard enough to get two people to agree on the same message, yet alone 40! How did this happen? This happened because even though men wrote down the words of the Bible, God himself wrote the Word of the Bible. Jesus Christ is the Word (John 1:1). He is the one who speaks to us. He is the one who created everything from nothing. The Bible is God's Word, his message to humanity written supernaturally by the Holy Spirit, the Spirit of Christ, through men. All 66 books in the Bible have the same message – a message of hope – a message of redemption. It starts with the story of creation and ends with the story of recreation. God is supernaturally and personally involved in his creation and in recreating us into who we were meant to be. The Bible is the book that gives us the information we need to understand what is going on in the world today, and how to embrace God's will.

The Bible is the book that will help you overcome your problems. The solutions to your problems are found in the very words of Jesus Christ. Your problem may exist in the physical realm, but your solution rests in the spiritual realm. I tried all kinds of solution, but only one solution works 100 % of the time: The Word of God! If I want to learn, for instance, about working out at the gym, I should read a book that will give insight into exercises that would help me get in shape. If I want to learn how to fix a broken-down appliance, I should Google it! But if I want to learn how to overcome my problems, how to know God's will, I must read the only book that will help me overcome – the Word of God. Think about it, the entire creation began with a simple statement: "Let there be light, and there was light" (Genesis 1:2). If all it took for the universe to be formed were words, think about how easy it would be to overcome your problem by power of God's Word!

As I stated earlier, the definition of insanity is doing the same thing over and over again expecting a different result. When you try and overcome your problems by your own power, you will fail. It takes a supernatural power to overcome. When God speaks, mountains move, and seas will part. Therefore, God's Word is available to knock down those mountains and divide those waters. When you speak the Word of God, you will get results! Overcoming your problem starts with the will, the will of God. When you embrace his will, you are embracing what is good and loving. When you embrace God's Word, you are embracing the very words of God, which can speak hope and power into your life. This message of hope starts in your brain, but then moves to your heart.

Songs have power because they move quickly from your brain to your heart. Songs are the words of the heart. When you sing a song, you are speaking words that penetrate the heart. This is why when you are in church singing songs, your attitude changes because you are singing the message of hope. When you listen to music, you move past your mind to your heart. The Psalmist writes, "I will sing praises to you Oh God" (Psalm 108:3). When you read or sing God's Word, you are changing your circumstances, because God's Word changes things. God's Word is what will change your situation, because God's

Word changes your mind. The Bible tells us that it is the Word of God that renews our minds (Romans 12:2).

When pilots fly planes, they usually let the plane fly on autopilot for a while. The directions are programmed into the computer, and the computer then flies the plane. Let's say that you are the pilot, and your plane is flying east on autopilot. You decide that you want to go west. You grab the controls and try to turn that plane around, but it won't turn. Why won't it turn? It won't turn because it is on autopilot. If you want to change directions, you have to reprogram the computer. If you want to change the way you think, your brain must be reprogrammed. You have to alter your autopilot. This can only happen when you reprogram it with a new operating system – the Word of God.

Thinking Problems

Some people have a drinking problem, but many people have a *thinking* problem. In fact, if you were to take the online survey called "Do I have a drinking problem?", and changed where it says *drinking* to *thinking,* you would be amazed to find out that thinking could be as destructive as drinking. Here are some of the questions (I have changed "drinking" to "thinking"):

- How often during the past year have you found out you were not able to stop thinking once you started?
- How often during the past year have you failed to do what was normally expected of you because of thinking?
- How often during the past year have you had feelings of guilt or remorse after thinking?

You can see that thinking can be a problem. Your thinking may be hindering your healing. The way you see things is directly related to your thinking. Are you a glass half-full person or a glass half-empty person? The real question is, do you even see the glass at all? In other words, most people are not grateful for having a glass to drink out of; they only see that the glass is half-empty or half-full. The best way to change your thinking is to become a grateful person. Grateful people realize that everything they have is a gift from God, even their problems. They don't let their problems control them, because they trust in a God who is working in their midst and is in control, a God who loves them and knows what is best for them. The only way you can overcome your problem is to get to know the one who can change your thinking. He is found in the pages of the Bible. When you read about God's will in the pages of his Word, you will become grateful because you will see that God can do miracles. He is the only one who can solve your problems, and the answers to your problems are found in his Word, the Bible.

Embrace God's Work

Solving your problems starts with faith, faith in a God who is actively working in your life. Jesus tells us that the most important work we can do is this: To believe in the one he has sent (John 6:29). Everything else we do should be based on faith in Christ. Whatever problems we have are nothing compared to the faith God has given us to believe. Believing in God is the beginning of embracing God's will for your life. In order to do this, I must embrace his work for my life.

The disciples who were with Jesus saw him do incredible things. He raised the dead, healed the sick, and cast out demons. All the while, Jesus was desirous that his disciples would believe to the point where they could do the same type of things. Although they eventually did do these miracles and more, they at first did not have enough faith to believe they could. This is why Jesus told them that even if they had faith as small as a mustard seed they could move mountains (Matthew 17:20). You see, believing in a God who can do miracles does not necessarily mean that you believe he will. I might have head-knowledge but not heart-knowledge.

Miracles are Around the Corner

When I was going through the illness described in this book, I never stopped believing God could do a miracle. The issue wasn't whether he *could* do it; the issue was whether he *would*. There's a huge difference between belief that is dormant and belief that is active. A belief that is active believes that God *can* do miracles. When we prayed for my dad's leg, we did not know whether he *would* heal his leg, but we always believed he *could* heal his leg. If you don't believe in a God who can do miracles, then your God is not big enough! For me, the issue has never been *if* God can solve my problems; it is more an issue of *whether* he will. And since I believe in a God who loves me, I believe that he knows what is best for me at each appointed time. Therefore, his timing and answer is what is best.

The hardest part of all this is the waiting. Waiting on God is hard because there are so many unanswered questions. If only he would tell me how this would all work out, then I would trust him. But then that would not be faith, and without faith, it's impossible to please God. When you are in the waiting room of life, never stop believing because God can do miracles. God may allow circumstances and problems to come into our lives for the very reason of building up our faith. When we get to the other side of the problem and are able to see the outcome, our faith will grow. This is the hope we have in Christ. We embrace God's will as we embrace his work in our lives, because your miracle could be just around the corner.

My time in rehab ended in November 2005, and I started to live a life of healing and recovery. I attended twelve-step meetings every day, sometimes twice a day. I reached out to people for help, something I would not have done before. I was learning to live a new life, a life based on the Bible, and on the support and help of others. This did not mean I was cured. It was a long, hard road. And what made things harder was that in 2006 I developed a stomach ailment that eventually landed me in the hospital for surgery. It seemed like things were getting worse, not better. The stomach surgery did not go as planned, and I developed more complications which led to more pain and more depression. This time, however, I was not going to lean on pills. I was going to lean on God, and on prayer. I reached out to anyone who would listen. I was not going to be prideful anymore. I realized that I would either embrace this new life, or I would die. God was faithful.

Soaring Like An Eagle

While driving on the toll road during these dark days, I would see eagles flying overhead. I live in a part of Orange County that still has open land and wilderness. These eagles were flying so high and looked so gracious and majestic. It was at this time that I pleaded with God, "Please, God, make me fly like that." That's when I heard a still small voice say, "David, one day soon, you will fly like that eagle." I held on to that promise and wouldn't let go. When sleepless, painful nights came, I would audibly say, "But Lord, you promised I would soar." When things seemed hopeless, I would remember this promise. And I would remember what someone told me, "Don't give up, your miracle may be just around the corner."

I'll never forget the Sunday our church moved from a local high school to our own building. On this Sunday, I decided to take our entire congregation outside to pray as we followed the Lord to our new home. We had met in that high school every Sunday for five years, and not once did I notice the words and painting on the side of the gym where we met. But that Sunday, I saw it! There it was... a painting of an eagle with the words, "Fly like an eagle"! That was God speaking to me! The time had come. I made it through. I graduated! From that moment on, my strength began to return, and my pain started to subside. I don't know why it was that particular Sunday that God chose to release me and allow me to start to fly, but he did. It was still a gradual glide until I would fly, but eventually I did. I can honestly say that what he said came true. My miracle happened. I now have a new perspective. I see things from 5,000 feet rather than from the ground. Challenges still prevail, and I still have problems, but I can see things differently now. Why? God revealed himself to me through my problems. If I didn't experience the pain, I would not recognize the relief. I had to travel through the desert to reach the promised land.

Paul's Thorn

Have you ever asked the question, "Lord, why do I have this problem?" If so, then you're in good company, because the Apostle Paul asked this same question. If you don't know about Paul and how much he accomplished for God, then I'm just going to tell you this: He accomplished more in a short ten years than most people accomplish in a lifetime. Everything he accomplished was accomplished while dealing with incredibly challenging problems. Problems like: being shipwrecked, beaten, mocked, and imprisoned. He experienced loss, pain, and abandonment. But maybe the most difficult problem he dealt with was what is known as "Paul's Thorn". Paul had a "thorn in his flesh". He wrote about this in his second letter to the Corinthian Church, found in the Bible. He said, "Three times I pleaded with the Lord to take it away from me" (2 Corinthians 12:8). No one knows for sure what this "thorn" was. Some think that he suffered from an eye disease because of the blindness that came upon him after seeing the risen Christ. Others say that this "thorn" was a symbol of the conflicts and challenges he had with those in the churches he planted. We do know that it was a thorn in his "flesh", so it must have had something to do with his body, maybe some kind of chronic pain. Whatever it was, it was problematic enough to mention in his letter to the church. Now, it is one thing to have a problem, it is another thing to have it *forever*. This seems to be the case with Paul's thorn.

As we read on, we find that God did not take away Paul's problem. Instead, God gave Paul extra grace to live with his problem. In verse 9, we read, "But he (God) said to me, 'my grace is sufficient for you, for my power is made perfect in weakness.'" What kind of answer is that?! I mean, this is the Apostle Paul praying, "Lord, please take away my pain," and how does God answer? "Paul, the problem is there for a purpose, so that you will rely on me more." Paul embraced God's will for his life, and this is what he received? Did Paul stop serving God? NO! Paul served him even more! Why? It was because Paul knew God. He knew that God would not allow something unless he had a specific reason and purpose. He knew that God's power was made perfect in Paul's weakness (1 Corinthians 12:9). Paul went through incredibly challenging problems, but all the while he kept serving and trusting God. This is what I'm talking about. This is what it means to embrace God's will for your life. Paul knew that he was not the only person who was dealing with problems. In fact, he knew that Jesus Christ dealt with even greater problems, but kept going, kept serving, even unto death. Paul did die, but I'm sure he heard these words, "Well done good and faithful servant."

The Storm

There's a story in the Bible found in Mark chapter 4. It's a story about a boat ride that caused extreme fear to come over Jesus's disciples. In verse 35, we find Jesus telling his disciples to get in the boat so that they could "go over to the other side." Somewhere in the middle of the sea, a furious storm rose up. The waves from the storm were so big that they poured in over the boat. The disciples were frantic, looking for Jesus. Do you know where they found Jesus? In the back of the boat asleep! Now, I don't know about you, but if Jesus asked me to get into a boat, and then I found him asleep while I was in peril, I would be more than slightly upset! The disciples felt this same way. They woke Jesus up and said to him, "Don't you even care if we drown?" Now think about that for a moment. Were they drowning? No, they were not. When the storms of life come upon us, and the waves seem like they are going to take us under, we get frantic. We start thinking the worse: "I'm going to drown", "My kids are going to end up in a bad place", "My husband or wife is going to leave me", "I'll never be able to get out from under this debt", "I'll have this thorn forever." The problem with all those statements is that they are not necessarily true, at least not at that moment. The disciples were not drowning, yet they said they were. Your husband or wife is not leaving you, though you think he or she is. Your kids are not running away from home yet, that's what you think is going to happen. This is the problem with our thoughts. Our thoughts can take us down faster than the storm! Jesus did end up calming the storm, and asked "Why are you so afraid? Do you still not have faith?" You see, the problem was not the storm; the problem was their lack of faith in the midst of the storm. I like a song written by Scott Krippayne. The lyrics say, "Sometimes he calms the storm, but sometimes he calms the child."² In other words, sometimes God will calm the storm, but other times he may choose to calm the child in the midst of the storm. This is the outcome of faith – you will remain calm even in the midst of the storms of life.

There's one more thing to realize about this story. The disciples got into the boat as they were told. But they missed a very important statement Jesus made to them: "Let us go over to the other side." Jesus told them they were going over to the other side, but when the storm rose, they forgot this important statement. The Bible tells us that God's Word never returns without accomplishing its purpose (Isaiah 55:11). Therefore, when Jesus told his disciples that they were going to the other side, they were going to the other side! No storm, no waves, no wind, no problem was going to stop them from going to where God wanted to take them. It is the same with you. When you believe in Jesus Christ and His Word, you believe in a God who can, at just a word, accomplish his purpose for you. He will get you to the other side no matter what! You may experience scary storms, devastating winds, deluging waves, but if Jesus says you're going to the other side, you are going there no matter what! It may take longer than you expect, the waves may be bigger than you'd like, but if you keep your eyes on Jesus and not on the storm, you will be calm because you will realize that Jesus is not asleep. He is just taking his time, because he knows that the storm you are in has a purpose, to grow your faith.

Abraham: Living By Faith

The Bible starts out with the account of creation. God created the world and everything in it in six days, and on the seventh day, he rested from his work. After creating man and woman, he let them have free will and walk in the garden with God. But the man and woman decided to rebel against God by rebelling against his word: "Do not eat of the tree of knowledge of good and evil" (Genesis 2:17). All Adam and Eve knew at the time was what was good. In fact, during God's creation, God said, "it is good" numerous times. The only time he said that it was not good was when he saw Adam alone. He then created Eve so that Adam would not be alone and that everything would be good again.

So when God told Adam and Eve to not eat from the tree of the knowledge of good and evil, he was trying to protect them from seeing the opposite of good: bad. He told them that if they ate of that tree, they would die. Why? It was because they would choose evil over good and therefore die. Death was never in the program. Death came because of sin. Sin is rebellion against God and His Word. When Adam and Eve ate of the forbidden fruit, they rebelled against the very Word and Will of God. This act of rebellion caused a huge problem: Sin had now entered the human race. The middle letter of

Sin is "I" because sin is about me, not about God. Sin is neglecting the very one who created you. Thank God that he had a plan – the plan was for His one and only Son to enter the human race and die on a cross for my sins. He took my place on the cross so I would not have to die, I could live! Jesus died in my place! This is the message of the Bible – that God loves the world so much that he sent his Son to die in my place, that whoever believes in him will not die, but have eternal life (John 3:16). Those who have faith in Christ will live!

Abraham exhibited Christ-like faith. He appears in Genesis chapter 12. Abraham was a descendent of Noah. His name was Abram, and he lived in a land called "Ur." At a young age, God spoke to Abram and said, "Go from your country, your people and your father's household, to the land I will show you" (Genesis 12:1). The story of Abraham is the story of him doing just that. But it was not easy, to say the least. It's never easy to leave everything behind and follow God. But God had given Abraham a promise, and Abraham believed God even though the road would be difficult. Abraham's road included leaving his family, his friends, and eventually doing something so incredibly difficult that because of this one act, God blessed Abraham beyond what he could even imagine.

Leaving the World Behind

In the summer of 1996, I left the safety of my surroundings to take a position at a church in Houston, Texas. I joke when I say that I prayed for humility, and God thought I said humidity and sent me to Texas! I was excited about this move, but my wife was not. She was not ready to venture out yet, but we both knew it was what God wanted us to do. We put the house on the market, but it did not sell before I had to leave. Therefore, I left my family behind to start working in Texas. It took three months for them to finally join me in Texas. Those three months were the hardest three months of my life. I remember feeling the pull so strong to go back to my wife and kids that I almost gave up and left. It was only by the prayers and support of my new friends in Texas that I stayed. I tell you this because following God can be very challenging. In fact, Jesus tells us that before we start following him, we should count the cost (Luke 14:28). But he also tells me that anyone who leaves houses and family to follow him will be tremendously blessed (Matthew 19:29). I have experienced so many incredible blessings by following Christ, but it has not been easy. I have learned that following Christ is challenging, but the blessings outweigh the difficulties by a lot. If you follow Christ to where he wants you to go, if you embrace his will for your life, you will meet people you never would have met and go places you would never have gone, and do things you would have never done. This is the great blessing for those who are faithful.

Abraham was a man of faith. He was faithful. Even in the midst of challenging circumstances, Abraham persevered. God asked him to travel to a land he did not even know of. Abraham left his family and home and followed God. During his following, he came upon challenges, including a time where he almost lost his wife and his life. During Abraham's walk with God, he was given a promise from God that he would one day become the father of a huge nation. In fact, God changed Abram's name to Abraham. Abram means, "father" but Abraham means, "father of many." Here is the problem: Abraham and his wife Sarah didn't have any children, and they could not have any children. That's a huge problem! Especially when you're supposed to be the father of a new nation. And especially when you're really old.

How can one become a father if he can't have kids? Abraham and Sarah realized this problem and tried to solve it on their own. They tried to handle things their way, rather than trust and wait on God's way. This only creates more problems. Abraham, at the request of his wife Sarah, slept with Sarah's handmaiden, and bore a son. This son, Ishmael, became great, but was not the son God promised.

Imagine that you are Abraham or Sarah. How would you handle your problem? Well, Abraham and Sarah moved ahead of God's will; and therefore, created a bigger problem. The problem was manifested through Ishmael. You see, Ishmael became a father of a nation, but this nation would be a constant enigma in the side of Abraham's nation. Even to this day, Ishmael is a thorn in the side of Israel. This is what happens when we try and solve our problems in our own wisdom and strength. We create more problems. Embracing God's will means waiting for God's solution, not your own.

When Abraham was in his 90's and Sarah in her 80's, God told them that they would finally have a son. They didn't believe at first, in fact Sarah laughed at this news. Imagine if this was what you were told. How would you react? Eventually, Isaiah was born. Isaiah is God's promised son. Isaiah became the father of Jacob, whose name was changed to Israel, and the rest is history. Isaiah was a miracle child. He was born to parents beyond their childbearing age. This means God had to do a miracle in Abraham and Sarah's bodies. This is what God does. His will happens in his time, and nothing can stop his will from happening, not even a dead body!

Everything was going great for Abraham and Sarah. They had finally settled down a bit and started a family. This meant that the promise would be fulfilled. That was until God told Abraham to do something incredibly unusual. He told Abraham to take his son, his one and only son, go up a mountain, and sacrifice him to the Lord. Imagine if God told you to do this? Imagine if you finally received your miracle, and then you were told to take your miracle, kill it, and give it back to God. This is what God said to Abraham. And guess what? Abraham obeyed God. But the good news is that God intervened and saved the promised child. You can read about it in Genesis chapter 22. This very act, the act of giving Isaac as a sacrifice, was enough to reveal Abraham's love and obedience to God. He was now ready to receive God's promise in all its fullness. In fact, God will often take us into a challenging situation to test our faith. He wants to see if we have more allegiance to the promise or to him. Nothing should ever take the place of God in your life. When God reveals a vision, he will take us on a journey to make us into the vision. This is how we grow and mature; this is how we learn to embrace God's will for our lives.

The Record Deal

My entire life, I dreamed of attaining a record contract. I wanted to write and record songs and make a living off this endeavor. Although I had some opportunities before I became a Christian, they never panned out. In 1997, I recorded a CD that landed on the desk of a major record executive. This executive expressed interest and told my producer that he was ready to sign me. One month later, his house burned down, and he lost interest. This devastated me. I was so ready to receive my dream that I flew to Nashville to try and meet with the record executive, only to experience a closed door after closed door.

I ultimately realized, after a few years, that not attaining the record deal was a good thing. If I had signed a record deal, I would have had to travel for much of the year. I would be away from my wife and kids, and miss them growing up. Even though my dream had died, I knew that God had a better plan. Because of not being constrained to a contract, I could encounter the blessings of seeing my children grow up; and for this I am grateful. This is often the case. We have our dreams, our desires, but sometimes these are the very things that can remove us from the things that are most important. We must take them up the mountain and give them back to him. Trusting God and his will is always best. Closed doors can be an opening for God's blessing.

Years after this incident, I was approached by a friend who had recently encountered an evening that changed his life. While attending a dinner for a local ministry, God spoke to him in a huge way. After the dinner, a video was played featuring a group of people who were very different than us. These people lived in a country called Sudan, in Africa. They were Christians, and because they were Christians, they were being excessively persecuted and slaughtered. He felt compelled to do something. Being a musician and recording artist, he decided to record a CD that would help raise awareness and finances for these persecuted Christians. He contacted me asking if I would donate a song to his project. The song I donated was "Make Me Your Voice," a song I wrote shortly after coming to Christ in 1992. This song is a prayer asking God to use my hands, my feet, and my voice to make a difference in the world. God blessed this project by joining us to a well-established record company. The record company heard my song, and decided to name the entire CD after my song, "Make Me Your Voice – A Voice for the Voiceless." I finally got a record contract! But this record contract was different. I would not make any money off my song, since I had donated the royalties for the benefit of the persecuted Church. This was fine with me, since my goal was not to exalt myself, but to exalt God and his purpose, "Lord, use my hands, use my feet, use my hands...." And he did!

The moral to this story is this: God's will WILL be done; but it won't always turn out the way I think it will. Abraham and Sarah tried to make things happen, and all they did was cause more problems. When they finally had a son, it looked a lot different than what they might have thought. Once I finally received a record contract, it looked a lot different than I thought. The key to embracing God's will for your life is accepting his will, not in the way you want it, but in the way he gives it.

Acceptance

In the Big Book (the book used for alcoholics anonymous), on page 417, you will read these words: *"Acceptance is the answer to all my problems today. When I am disturbed, it is because I find some person, place, thing, or situation – some fact of my life – unacceptable to me, and I can find no serenity until I accept that person, place, thing, or situation as being exactly the way it is supposed to be at this moment. Nothing, absolutely nothing, happens in God's world by mistake."*[3] Think about the peace you can have by just following these simple orders. Acceptance doesn't mean that you have to passively sit there and accept without trying to get help; the kind of acceptance that brings peace translates to one word: Trust. *"Lord, I trust you, even when it doesn't make sense. I trust you for the outcome, because I know that you have my best interest at heart. Even though this is hard for me, I accept knowing that you are not finished yet. You are just beginning. You are caring for me, comforting me, and correcting me. I have decided to trust you; therefore, I accept your medicine and will take it."*

Those words helped me through many a dark day. I knew that things were happening for a reason. I would discuss my problems with people who would not try to fix my problems, but would just listen. I would suit up and show up. Even when I didn't feel like going, I would go. I learned that I could not continue to do life alone. I must do my part, and let God do his. I must realize that even if it doesn't seem so, God is working. He is accomplishing his will. He is a loving God who is giving me what I need. I can either accept his gift or reject it. When I reject God's gift, I am rejecting God's will. This leads to more problems than the ones I already had. Notice that the author of the above statement says, "Nothing, absolutely nothing, happens in God's world by mistake." I don't know if the man who wrote those words is a Christian. What I do know is that he has the proper view of who God is. I, being a Christian, believe in a God who, at his very spoken word, changed the entire universe. What was once void and lifeless is now full of life. I am someone who continues to learn about God and about trusting him. I still struggle with trusting him. But at least I have learned to accept his will as something good, no matter what it looks like through the lens of this world. God's will, his word, and his work, are accomplishing things that can only be experienced through faith. God is perfect, and he never makes mistakes.

Step 6: *F orgive*

"There are people in your life who've come and gone
They let you down and hurt your pride
Better put it all behind you; life goes on
You keep carryin' that anger, it'll eat you up inside"[1]
– Don Henley (Heart Of The Matter)

*I*n the 1980's, during an economic downturn, music gigs became sparse. Therefore, I had to look outside the music business to gain income. One job, which I hated, was working with a construction-worker friend. He hired my brother and I to help him demolish homes in the Riverside area. These homes were very old, and it wasn't until years later that I came to find out that they were ridden with asbestos. Asbestos is a fibrous material that is often used for building insolation. Asbestos is also highly carcinogenic and causes diseases such as mesothelioma. My friend who hired me was a marine who had just come home from the war in Grenada and was very unstable, to say the least. He had us working day and night tearing down and demolishing homes so the land could be sold to new owners. It was a difficult and taxing job. I couldn't wait to get back to the music business!

Our lives are like those homes. We get demolished by other people, destroyed by the words and actions of those whom we thought were friends. Our lives become ridden with the poison of unforgiveness, the cancer of resentment, which is much worse than asbestos. Unforgiveness eats at the core of your heart and soul. It is poison that eats away day-after-day, eventually killing you. We get hurt, and we hurt others in return. There's a saying that goes, "hurt people, hurt people." We hurt others because we have been hurt, but unforgiveness doesn't hurt the other person, it hurts us. Nothing hinders God's will for our lives more than unforgiveness. There's nothing that will hinder your healing more than unforgiveness, bitterness, and resentment.

Celebrities are Cool

Growing up with celebrities was cool, yet difficult. Jealousy abounds when you don't have what others have. One of those celebrities became my best friend. I met him in junior high, and he quickly became my best friend. I loved him like my brother, and I felt like his father and mother were my second father and mother. I would hang out at his house almost every day after school. We were best friends. Seeing my best friend become famous was hard for me. For my entire life, I wanted to prove to others, especially to my parents, that I was worth something. The fact that I could write songs and play music was important to my self-esteem. You would think that seeing my best friend become famous would be encouraging to me, but it wasn't. I was so insecure; seeing him become famous, and me not becoming famous, was discouraging, to say the least. I was filled with resentment. I hate to admit this, because it is embarrassing, but it was the truth. My resentment came to a boiling point the day I rode with him to a party celebrating his rise to stardom. He rented a limousine and invited me along. Again, you would think that riding in a limousine with a famous person would be one of the coolest things anyone could do. But for me, it wasn't. Why? Because that limousine should have been my limousine! At least that's how I felt. I was the one who worked the hardest. I was the one who got the gigs. I was the one who "discovered" him. Resentment eats away at your soul and at your relationships.

That night was the beginning of the end for us. I regret this so much, because for years after that, I held resentment towards him that caused me to never go over his house, never hang out, and never play music with him for a long time. He and I got in an argument that night based on my pride. It was nothing he did; it was all about me. It was all about what I thought I deserved. This is what jealousy, resentment, and unforgiveness does. It eats away at your friendships, your ego, and your pride. Unforgiveness is like poison, but the one who drinks it is the one who has it. Instead of the other person dying, we die. Unforgiveness is like drinking poison and waiting for the other person to die. Sadly, it is the one holding on to the unforgiveness who dies. This is why forgiveness is so important to your healing. God wants you to live. Living with unforgiveness is not living at all.

In this chapter I want to talk about three aspects of forgiveness: 1) <u>Forgiveness starts with me</u>. I have to be the one who forgives. I can't wait for others to apologize. My healing depends on me forgiving others as Christ forgave me. 2) <u>Forgiveness comes from God</u>. I can't forgive others the way Christ forgives me if I am not dependent on God to give me the strength to forgive. I have to rely on his grace to get me through each step of the way. 3) <u>Forgiveness flows through</u>

Christ. I can't forgive others if I have not accepted God's forgiveness through Christ. I must first receive God's forgiveness before I can truly forgive others.

Step 6: **Forgiv**e those who have hurt me and learn to forgive myself

Forgiveness Starts With Me

The nightclubs were getting darker and grosser. What I never saw before was what I was now seeing every night – the pain, the hurt, the disappointment, all showing up in a place that prides itself with providing "happy hours." There is nothing happy about happy hours! Well, unless they have half-price food! This is why Billy Joel coined the phrase, "he's sharing a drink he calls loneliness…making love to his tonic and gin."[2] What I had become familiar with was now becoming unfamiliar. I used to relate to these feelings, but now something was different. What was different? Forgiveness! I accepted God's forgiveness through his Son, Jesus Christ. But many of these people had not.

My favorite song to sing during this time was a song by Don Henley, called "Heart of the Matter." I can honestly say that this is one of the best songs ever written. The lyrics are incredible. They touch on what everyone wants and desires – forgiveness. When I would sing this song, the place would become silent. All the chatter, distractions, and unfocussed people would be pulled into an experience that is hard to explain in words. All I know is that after singing the song, I would have people approach me all night long asking,

"Will you please sing that song again?" Why did they want me to sing that song again? Because the Heart of the Matter is truly forgiveness, it is what we desire… what we long for. And the sad part is that most of the people in the club were there because they couldn't forgive themselves. Sure, some may have even accepted God's forgiveness; but for some reason, they were unwilling to allow forgiveness into their own life. I can tell you this because I was one of those people.

There was a little boy visiting his grandparents on their farm. He was given a slingshot to play with out in the woods. As he was practicing, he saw Grandma's pet duck. Just out of impulse, he let the slingshot fly, hit the duck square in the head, and killed it. In a panic, he hid the dead duck in the woodpile, only to notice his sister watching! Sally had seen it all, but she said nothing. After lunch the next day, Grandma said, "Sally, let's wash the dishes." But Sally said, "Grandma, Johnny told me he wanted to help in the kitchen." Then Sally whispered to him, "Remember the duck?" So Johnny did the dishes. Later that day, Grandpa asked if the children wanted to go fishing, and Grandma said, "I'm sorry, but I need Sally to help make supper." Sally just smiled and said, "Well, that's all right because Johnny told me he wanted to help." She whispered again to Johnny, "Remember the duck?" So Sally went fishing, and Johnny stayed to help. After several days of Johnny doing both his chores and Sally's, he finally couldn't stand it any longer. He came to Grandma and confessed that he had killed the duck.

Grandma knelt down, gave him a hug, and said, "Sweetheart, I know. I was standing at the window, and I saw the whole thing, and because I love you, I forgave you. I was just wondering how long you would let Sally make a slave of you."

When you won't or can't forgive yourself, you will become a slave to the unforgiveness and guilt in your heart. It will take over and become like poisonous asbestos. It will eat away at your mind, your heart, and your soul. Your life will begin to deteriorate, and eventually your joy and peace will die. You may not even know what's going on, because you have held on to this for so long.

I knew a lady who would not forgive her ex-husband. She started to become blind in one eye. No doctor could help her. One day, while in church, the preacher was preaching about the importance of forgiveness. She realized that she hadn't forgiven her ex-husband and also hadn't forgiven herself. Once she allowed forgiveness to permeate her soul, her eyesight came back. Yes, resentment and unforgiveness, even guilt, can cause physical illness. Realize that your body is made up of a soul, a mind, and a spirit. Your physical body is attached to each of the other parts. Therefore, when one part is sick, the other part suffers. You can't allow unforgiveness to take residence and think that it will not affect your entire being. You will become its slave, and you will miss out on the life God wants you to live.

Peter – the unforgiven disciple

One person in the Bible who had a hard time forgiving himself was Peter. Peter was one of Jesus' three most important disciples. It was Peter, James, and John, who had the opportunity see things that the others didn't see. They were in Jesus' inner circle. Peter was the one whom Jesus said would hold the keys to his Church. Yet Peter was also the one who denied Jesus three times causing him to weep bitterly and eventually go back to his fishing business. It was while Peter was fishing, after Jesus rose from the dead, when he finally experienced true forgiveness; when he was finally able to forgive himself.

The evening was coming upon them as they wrapped up their fishing excursion. It was then that someone appeared on the shore. The other disciples could not see who it was, but Peter knew. "It's Jesus!" Peter jumped out of the boat with all his clothes on and ran to Jesus! Peter was so happy. He even got to eat fish with his best friend. But it may have been about that time when Peter remembered, "I denied you, Jesus. I don't even deserve to be here with you." That was when Jesus began to ask Peter a series of questions. The questions were in regards to whether Peter loved Jesus. "Peter, do you love me?" to which Peter answered, "Yes, Lord, you know I love you." This exchange went on three times. Each time, I'm sure Peter must have felt worse. "Why is Jesus asking me this? Doesn't he know I already feel horrible about letting him down?" But Jesus kept asking. Each time Jesus would respond to Peter's positive response with "Peter, if you love me, feed my sheep, take care of my sheep."

Now, I'm not sure if what was happening here with Jesus had sunk in yet. Think about it. Peter had denied his Lord three times. And now Jesus had asked Peter three times, "do you love me?" Do you get it? Jesus asked Peter this question three times to show that he was forgiven. I mean, why would Jesus take the time to show up again after he rose from the dead? Why would he ask three specific questions of the same manner? Wouldn't it have been better for him to just go back to heaven from where he came? But Jesus had more work to do – he came back to Peter to help Peter not only know he was forgiven, but for Peter to truly forgive himself. Jesus even confirmed this by restoring his position back into the Church – "feed my sheep", which means to lead and teach Jesus' disciples with the

Word of God. It was after this when Peter finally got it. He preached a sermon, and three thousand people came to Christ! Peter began to change the world because he knew he was truly forgiven. The point is this: You can't change the world unless you're willing to be changed by God's forgiveness. The only way you can truly be changed is to truly accept God's forgiveness through his Son, Jesus Christ, and realize that no matter what you have done, or what you will ever do, is not greater than what Jesus did for you on the cross!

<u>Forgiveness Comes From God</u>

A woman bought a parrot for a pet. All the parrot did was to treat her badly. It insulted her, and every time she tried to pick it up, it would peck at her arm. The parrot continued to insult her day after day, saying things like, "You're ugly! I can't stand you!" And it pecked at her arm as she carried it. One day, she got fed up with the parrot, and as it was insulting her, she picked it up, opened the freezer door, and threw it in, slamming the door shut. From inside, the parrot was still going on for about five seconds, and then it was suddenly quiet. She thought, "Oh no, I killed it!" She opened the door, and the parrot just looked at her. She picked it up. Then the parrot said: "I'm very sorry. I apologize for my bad behavior and promise you there will be no more of that. From now on, I will be a respectful, obedient parrot." "Well OKAY" she said, "Apology accepted". The parrot said "Thank you". Then he said, "Can I ask you something?" She said, "Yes, What?" The parrot looked at the freezer, and asked, "What did the chicken do?"

Have you ever felt like the woman in this story? The insults just keep coming, and mostly from your own mind! Your thoughts can kill you! On the other hand, have you ever felt like that parrot? "Oh no, what did I do *now*?" "I'm never going to be forgiven for this one!" The people in those nightclubs… most of them felt like that. I used to feel like that too. "How could God ever forgive me for all the bad things I've done?" After I accepted God's forgiveness through his Son, Jesus Christ, I felt like a weight had been lifted from my shoulders. Why? It is because everyone, including me, needs forgiveness. There's a beautiful poem that goes like this…

> If our greatest need had been information,
> God would have sent us an educator;
> If our greatest need had been technology,
> God would have sent us a scientist;
> If our greatest need had been money,
> God would have sent us an economist;
> If our greatest need had been pleasure,
> God would have sent us an entertainer;
> But our greatest need was forgiveness,
> So, God sent us a Savior.
> -Anonymous

There's a Spanish story of a father and son who had become estranged. The son ran away, and the father set off to find him. He searched for months to no avail. Finally, in a last desperate effort to find him, the father put an ad in a Madrid newspaper. The ad read: "Dear Paco, meet me in front of this newspaper office at noon on Saturday. All is forgiven. I love you. Your Father." On Saturday, 800 Pacos showed up, looking for forgiveness and love from their fathers.

God, our Father, sent his only Son into the world so that we could receive forgiveness. All the bad things I have done in the past, all the bad things I will do today, and all the bad things I will do in the future, are all forgiven, not because of something I did, but because of something God did. God knew that I needed a Savior, someone to save me from my sins. Thank God I heard his voice and accepted his gift of forgiveness!

I have a friend who is a lifeguard. He tells me that the hardest people to save are the ones who are trying to save themselves. This is so true. I can imagine how the lifeguard feels when he goes into the water to save a drowning swimmer, only to have to fight against the swimmer's self-will that he is trying to save himself. This is the problem God has with us. We are always trying to save ourselves, and all the while we are only sinking deeper into the sea of unforgiveness. The Apostle Paul was this kind of person.

Forgiveness in the Desert

Imagine if the most evil person turned from his evil ways and started to follow Jesus Christ. Imagine if Hitler did this, or Osama Bin Laden. Imagine if all the terrorists in ISIS stopped terrorizing people and started living for Jesus Christ. This is exactly what happened in the Apostle Paul's life. Before he became Paul, everyone knew him as Saul. Saul was a devout orthodox Jew. He grew up in a devout Jewish home and went to school to study under the greatest teacher of Jewish law of the time – Gamaliel. If Saul were alive today, he would have received a PhD in Jewish religious studies. Saul was zealous for God and God's law. That was until he met Jesus in the desert.

It was a hot desert afternoon. Saul was traveling from Jerusalem to Damascus, Syria, with letters in his hand, letters giving him permission to arrest and detain anyone who followed "The Way." That was the name of those who were following Jesus – The Way. Suddenly he heard a loud noise and then saw a very bright light. The light was bright enough to blind him for three days! He fell off his horse only to hear a voice say to him, "Saul, Saul, why do you persecute me?" "Who are you, Lord?" Saul asked. "I am Jesus, whom you are persecuting" (Acts 9:5). Notice that even though Saul was not directly persecuting the person of Jesus Christ, he was persecuting the Body of Jesus Christ – His Church. This is risky business – persecuting the Church! Anyone who does this will be held to account. But Saul didn't know this until he heard the voice of his Lord speaking to him.

Notice Saul called the voice "Lord". Why would Saul call someone he didn't even know "Lord"? It must have been the sound of the voice – the power behind his voice. After all, this was the same voice that spoke the universe into creation. Saul's friends heard a sound, but didn't hear the voice. Why? Because it was Saul to whom Jesus spoke. It is important to understand that when Jesus speaks, and you hear his voice, you must listen. You must stop all you are doing, and ask, "What do you want, Lord?" This experience in the desert changed Saul's life forever. Jesus had an appointment with Saul, and Saul fell off his horse! God will cause you to fall off your horse sometimes, but don't worry… you will get back on. The horse might be the same horse you rode in on, but you will be a different person!

Saul finally came to, and his friends took him and cared for him. But for three days, Saul could not see. The last thing Saul saw was the face of Jesus. In the old days, one would take pictures with a camera that used film. Film was to be kept in the dark until developed. "What happened to Saul is a perfect picture of what happens in photography: Film, coated with light-sensitive salts and chemicals, is kept in darkness. When the shutter opens, light pours in, and whatever is seen in the light at that second is printed on the film. Then it's quickly returned to darkness, lest it be overexposed. Finally, it is taken into a darkroom, where it is placed in a chemical solution and fully developed. When Saul was persecuting Christians, he was in spiritual darkness. Suddenly, on the road to Damascus, the shutter release was pushed, and he saw the Light. Then he was returned to darkness through physical blindness in order for the image of Jesus alone to be permanently imprinted upon his heart and developed within his life."[3]

Saul's name is an interesting one. I'm sure he was named after the first king of Israel – who, by the way, failed miserably. Why did he fail? He failed because he did not do what God wanted him to do. He failed to keep God at the forefront of his mind. This Saul (Paul) was not going to make the same mistake! He changed his name from Saul to Paul. Saul means, "Asked of God". Paul means "humble" or "little" one. Saul, who thought he was great in God's eyes, became Paul (little) because he had a one-on-one encounter with the risen Christ! Saul was "Asked of God" to become Jesus Christ's ambassador and in order to do this Saul had become Paul, humble before God's sight. That is what happens to us too when we have this encounter with Christ. We realize how little we really are, and how great he truly is, but, what about Paul's former life? What about the murders he took part in of innocent believers? What about the way he persecuted God's church? As Paul would say, "Christ came into this world to save sinners – of whom I am the worst" (1 Timothy 1:15).

God's forgiveness is for everyone, even the worst of sinners. We have a saying at my church, "The Gate is a place for everyone, even you!" God accepts anyone and everyone who calls on the name of His Son, Jesus Christ. Paul became one of the most important people in the entire Bible. God used Paul to write most of the New Testament. Paul's life changed the moment he met Christ. He then went on to change millions of lives over the past 2,000 years who have read the words of God written on the pages of the Bible. Only God can do this. Only God can forgive your sins and set you on a new path. In fact, it was this very thing that caused Jesus so much trouble. He would walk up to people and say, "your sins are forgiven". The Jewish leaders would contest him, saying, "How do you forgive people's sins? For only God can forgive sins." This is exactly the point. Only God can forgive your sins, and it is God who does exactly that. Forgiveness comes from God through Christ.

Forgiveness Flows Through Christ

The crucifixion of Jesus was one of the most horrific deaths ever. I'm not going to go into detail regarding the physical torture that happens through crucifixion, but know this – No one should ever have to die this way. But it was in this way Jesus chose to die. Rome was known for its crucifixions. In fact, in around 40BC, in Rome, a historian recorded that 2,000 people were crucified in a single day solely for the entertainment purposes of the emperor.[4] Crucifixion was the means by which the Roman government enforced control; the fear of being crucified was enough to stifle crimes and governmental overthrow.

Jesus Christ died on that cross for our sins. He never sinned yet took on my (and your) sins so that you could be set free, so that you could have 24/7 access to God. Remember that God is holy; he is unapproachable for he is *the* king. Yet, because of the forgiveness of sins offered by Jesus Christ through the cross, he gives us continuous access because now we are forgiven; we are seen as righteous (right with God) when we are "in" Christ. One becomes "In Christ" the moment they place their faith in him for their eternal salvation. Once this happens, God's Spirit comes into one's life and makes them "born-again" – Born from above. This is this very reason that one can now have access to the creator of the universe. It is not something that you could ever do – only God could do this. Only God can forgive your sins and make you new. The problem is that most people never take advantage of the gift God offers through his Son. It would be like never opening the gifts you receive on Christmas. They are there, under the tree, but you are unwilling to open them. Why would you not open the gift of salvation through forgiveness? Hopefully you have received this free gift by now. If not, re-read chapter 2 (Step 2: Believe), and take this very important step towards healing. I promise you that you will not experience physical healing if you won't be healed spiritually. It is spiritual healing that is most important, because it is our spirit that will be renewed the moment you believe in Jesus Christ. You will be transformed and made new.

During Jesus' life here on earth, he said many provocative things. One of these statements came during a very important Jewish holiday, the Feast of Tabernacles. The Feast or Tabernacles was when Israel commemorated those who were delivered from slavery in Egypt to freedom through the Red Sea. Because they lived in the wilderness, they had to dwell in tents (tabernacles). God provided water for them through a rock. This rock, as the Apostle Paul states, was the spiritual presence of Jesus Christ (1 Corinthians 10:4). On the last day of this great feast, Jesus stood in the street and told everyone, *"Let anyone who is thirsty come to me and drink. Whoever believes in me, as*

Scripture has said, rivers of living water will flow from within them" (John 7:37). In saying this, he was stating that he, like that rock in the wilderness, is the source of spiritual water and sustenance. This spiritual healing would happen to those in whom he would release his Spirit (the Holy Spirit) given to those who would believe in him. He was saying, that through him, eternal life flows and forgiveness is given. On another day, Jesus said this: *"Whoever drinks the water I give them will never thirst. Indeed, the water I give them will become in them a spring of water welling up to eternal life"* (John 4:14). He said this to a woman who was very thirsty.

A Noontime Appointment With Jesus

Have you ever been so thirsty that you could hardly take it? When my father was ill, he could not drink water from a glass. He could only take little sips of ice as we held the ice-cube up to his mouth. I felt so bad for him. No one ever wants to feel this thirsty and not be able to be quenched. However, many people are thirsty for spiritual water, yet live life sipping on ice cubes rather than drinking from a deep well of nourishment. This was the plight of the woman at the well. She had been married five times and was living with her sixth husband. That, in itself, no matter what you think about divorce, shows a longing for something, doesn't it? I mean if you have been married six times, maybe it's time to start looking in the mirror, or better yet, looking outside yourself to find satisfaction. I worked with a very famous recording artist and performer who had been married eight times! I always wondered if his eighth marriage would last; and to this day, he is still married. Maybe he learned. I wonder if people who have been married this many times start to wonder if the problem of staying married is their problem, or if they still think it is the other person? For the woman at the well, she was thirsty, but not for water, she was thirsty for love, true love.

Jesus, being a Jewish man, would never find himself sitting with a woman like this woman. She was a Samaritan – half Jewish, half something else. Samaritans were judged as unclean; and no one, especially a devout Jewish man, should sit with her and talk with her. Yet, Jesus went out of his way to sit with her. He traveled the long way home just so he could meet with her. He had an appointment with her at noon at a well. This well was where women would come and draw water for their family, but not usually during the mid-day sun. God had orchestrated all this so he could reach a very thirsty woman, and so we could read about this encounter thousands of years later. Why? It is because there is an important message of forgiveness in this conversation. The woman came to draw physical water; Jesus came to give her spiritual water. The woman quickly realized there was something different about this man; he spoke of a well that would never run dry. He wasn't speaking of the well she drew from, but rather the well deep in her soul. Her well was empty and she was not well. She had given all she had, and didn't have anymore to give. Jesus saw this need, and he met her need by revealing to her that He was the only person who could ever fill the hole in her heart, her spiritual thirst. The water of her soul had run dry and the hole was deep, but Jesus can fill holes with spiritual water that meets your deepest need.

What about a sin like this?

Have you ever felt like you'd gone too far? Committed a sin that was unforgiveable? I felt like that all the time. It is amazing now to know that all those sins have been forgiven. If I were God, I would think twice before forgiving some of the sins I committed. I was ashamed at things I did, especially when hurting other people. We hurt God all the time, yet he is ready to forgive. This is amazing! Thank God for his forgiveness.

One woman in the Bible felt like I did. She was caught in the very act of adultery. She was marched half-naked, and thrown on the floor in front of a crowd of judgmental, hypocritical people. There was no secret to the fact that anyone who was caught having sex outside of marriage would be stoned. That was the law, and everyone knew the law and took the law seriously. Jesus was the only one who could challenge the law, because as the Bible says, he fulfilled all of God's laws (Matthew 5:17). As he looked at this shamed woman, he knew what he had to do. He challenged the crowd by saying, *"he who has not sinned, cast the first stone"* (John 8:7).

Think about that statement. If you were in the crowd, how would you have reacted? Put yourself in this crowd, and think of yourself as a devout religious Jew, who tried very hard to keep the law. Here before you, was someone who broke the law. What would you do? How would you react to Jesus' statement? I can tell you that hearing Jesus' words would have shaken my world. I can't even imagine hearing this and not being convicted of all the bad things I had done and thought. Every wrong thought, feeling, and action, would have passed before my eyes like a bad movie. This is why the crowd disbanded, one by one. Now it was only Jesus and the woman. "Has anyone condemned you?" "No one, sir", she answered. To which Jesus responded, "Go now and sin no more" (John 8:11).

Remember, this was God standing there looking at her. She was guilty and had no excuse. Yet Jesus chose to forgive her sins. I believe, however, this was all a set-up. For instance, where was the man? It takes two to tango, if you know what I mean! I believe these hypocrites wanted to test Jesus as to how he would handle someone who broke the law, so they grabbed this woman like a lamb left out to slaughter. Jesus, though, knew that sin is sin. Whether you commit adultery or tell a lie, it is all categorized as sin, because sin is breaking the law. If I get a speeding ticket, I might be careful for a while. However, if I don't get caught again, I will keep speeding. If I get caught, I might stop speeding for maybe a month, but then I will go back to breaking the law. This is what we do. We keep sinning, and when we get caught, we say, "I promise to never do that again", yet it's only a matter of time until we break the law again by doing the same behavior over and over. This woman broke the law, but was set free. Why? Because God is the one who forgives, and it is Jesus from whom God's forgiveness flows. "Go and sin no more." Why? Because sin matters! Sin is serious. Jesus died on a cross for our sins. When we diminish sin to something less than it is, we are diminishing the power of the cross and what it means. In fact the Bible says that anyone who says they do not sin is a liar (1 John 1:8). Remember, admitting you are a sinner who needs a Savior, is the first step to healing. This woman, I believe was healed, because God set her free.

Forgiveness Has No Ends

Good Friday is when we remember what Jesus did for us on the cross. We should remember what he did every day, but it is on Good Friday when the Church usually has a special service commemorating this incredible act of love. While Jesus was on the cross, he could see his accusers and hear their insults, yet he was willing to say, *"Father, forgive them, for they do not know what they are doing"* (Luke 23:34). Forgiveness is a choice. Jesus chose to forgive you. He didn't have to forgive. He chose to forgive. As he died on that cross for you and me, he heard a voice next to him say, "Jesus, remember me when you come into your kingdom" (Luke 23:32). It was the voice of a thief. There were actually two thieves, one on either side. One thief chose to spend his final moments alive mocking Jesus, the other decided to trust in Jesus. People who continuously mock Jesus will never experience healing and forgiveness.

I believe in deathbed conversions, because this thief was on his deathbed. Yet, instead of mocking Jesus like the other thief, he spoke of his faith in Jesus. I'm sure he knew who Jesus was, because he spoke of the kingdom. God's kingdom was what Jesus spoke of all the time. The thief knew his time was short and asked for forgiveness. How did Jesus respond? Jesus answered, *"Truly I tell you: today you will be with me in paradise"* (Luke 23:43). Jesus, an innocent man, was able to forgive a guilty man and invite him to be with him in heaven. This is so incredibly amazing to me. A sinless God would forgive a sinful human, a thief. I am like that thief. Not because I stole something... well, actually I did steal some sunglasses when I was young, but compared to everything else I did, that was minor. I am like that thief because I deserve death. I broke the law. I stole from God. Yet God chose to forgive me. Why? He forgives me because I believe in Him. That's all. I did not work or earn God's forgiveness for that I cannot do; all I did was place my faith in Jesus Christ, God's Son. I don't just believe *about* him; I believe *in* him. I made a decision to place my eternal salvation in the hands of a crucified God. But you know the rest of the story – he is not dead, he's alive! I can know that he will do what he promises, because he is alive. I believe in a risen Jesus Christ, because I saw him and heard his voice, maybe not with my physical eyes but with the spiritual eyes he gave me. He opened my eyes so I could see and receive God's forgiveness. And I believe that he is able to do more than I can even ask or imagine. I hope that you will believe and receive God's forgiveness too.

Forgiveness Is a Two-Way Street

My relationship with God goes two directions: vertical and horizontal. God's forgiveness is a vertical forgiveness. He forgives all my sin and invites me to heaven with him. It is a one-way forgiveness. But horizontal forgiveness (human forgiveness) is a two-way street, and God expects me to live both vertically and horizontally. Human forgiveness goes two ways – *to* others and *from* others. When I sin against another human, I must ask for forgiveness *from* the other person (apologize); and when someone sins against me, I must offer forgiveness *to* the other person, even when they don't apologize. This is the subject matter we will delve into next.

Forgiveness From Others

Out of the twelve steps of Alcoholics Anonymous, three of them deal with making amends and asking forgiveness from others. Why are one-fourth of the twelve steps attributed to asking forgiveness of others? Because much of our destructive behavior can be traced back to feelings of guilt and shame associated with harming God and others. For instance, an alcoholic or drug addict will often continue to drink because the feeling of guilt is so strong that they just need relief, which they find in a bottle or in a drug. Until this unhealthy chain is broken, the addict will never heal. Guilt is the cause of many problems, including physical and emotional sickness and pain. Psychiatrists say that 70% of the people in the hospital could leave today if they knew how to resolve guilt and move on. When we swallow our guilt, our stomach keeps score. My stomach was so bad, that I had to have surgery to repair it. If only I could be like the thief on the cross and enter into paradise the moment I'm forgiven. But no! I had to hold on to unforgiveness, because guilt and shame were my friends. I stated earlier that healing only happens when we are willing to admit we are wrong. This also means that I must admit when I'm wrong in holding on to guilt and shame because those two friends are no friends at all! They are my enemies. They are like the duck and the parrot. They keep me from experiencing the joy of eternal life. Jesus came to give us a full life, which starts the moment you receive his forgiveness, but we want to hold on to the guilt, resentment, and shame, instead of leaving them there on the cross. Why do we do this? One word: Feelings!

I loved the song, "Feelings" by Morris Albert. You may not have heard this song, but the melody and lyrics are great. Feelings, however, should not enter into the discussion about doing the right thing. Feelings should just stay in a song. Once we allow feelings to dictate our thoughts and actions, we get into trouble. Feelings are just that – feelings. Feelings come and go. If I judge who I am based on feelings, I would feel like a no-good, guilty, shameful sinner. That is exactly what the Devil wants me to feel like. But God says something different. God says I am forgiven. I can't heal if I am unwilling to admit when I am wrong. Make a decision today to stop letting your feelings run your life, and instead let God's truth run your life!

The reason I can ask forgiveness from others is the same reason God has forgiven me. I asked and he responded. This does not mean that everyone will forgive me. I can only do my part; it is up to the other person to do theirs. Thank God that he is faithful to forgive when I admit I am wrong! It is not the case with everyone else. But that is okay. I have to be able to keep my side of the street clean. I can't have garbage built up on my lawn because it gets in the way of experiencing peace. If I don't do my part by admitting when I am wrong, the garbage will be piled high!

There are many times when I have to ask people for forgiveness. It is called *apologizing*! To apologize means to admit you are wrong. The word "apologize" comes from the Greek word, "apologia", which means to "make an excuse or defense." The Apostle Paul would often defend his faith in Christ in front of others; he would make an excuse for why he believed what he believed. In its original context, it is a judicial term. A good lawyer will "apologize" for why he believes the person is innocent. We get the Christian term, "apologetics" from this word, which means to present a defense for our faith in Christ. To apologize to someone for something we have done wrong is not a defense for why we did it, or an excuse... it is to admit that we are wrong. We defend our wrongness, which means we present an argument for why we are wrong. The worst way to approach apologizing is to give excuses and blame others for our mistake. That is what we call immature behavior. That is the behavior of a two-year old. We, as adults, should make a defense as to why we are wrong, not make excuses or blame others for our mistakes or for why the other person is wrong. "I'm sorry for treating you badly", "It was wrong of me to lie to you." Those are the words of a mature, "on-their-way to healing" person. Whatever the wrong, it should be defended from a point of view that we take responsibility for our wrong. This is the proper way to apologize. What if it is not all your fault? Still, you must apologize for your part of it. Many times, when apologizing, I know that it is not all my fault, but for the health of the relationship, and mostly for my spiritual and emotional health, I must take responsibility for my part of the problem. I can't stress enough the importance of this. In order to heal, I must apologize when I am wrong, and give others the opportunity to offer forgiveness.

Forgiveness To Others

Asking forgiveness of others is the easy part; offering forgiveness to others is hard! But if you are unwilling to forgive, you will remain sick! The main reason I stayed so sick for so long was due to my unwillingness to forgive. I held on to anger, which grew into a huge depression. If you struggle with depression, there may be a root (or roots) of unforgiveness. I encourage you to be willing to forgive, because being unwilling will only lead to a deeper and deeper depression. I was sick and tired of being sick and tired. I hope you will allow God to forgive you, and allow yourself to forgive others.

The reason I use the word, "unwilling" when speaking of the act of forgiveness, is because, like love, forgiveness is a choice. I can't tell you how many times I didn't feel like forgiving someone, but I can't rely on my feelings. I have to make a choice. What if someone does something that is unforgiveable? I have heard of some incredible painful stories. When I hear of child-abuse, or sex-slavery, or any kind of abuse on innocent young victims, my first reaction is to send them to the electric chair. Hitler was one of the most evil people to ever live. ISIS is beheading people just because they are different than them. Think about how incredibly painful this is, not only to the person, but also to the person's family. Recently there was a story in Ohio of a few women who were kidnapped, tied up, and sexually abused for over ten years! Can you imagine the resentment and anger of the girls and also their family? Yet, I heard the girls say things like, "I choose to forgive." Why did they choose to forgive? Because they know that holding on to the past will hinder them from moving forward. Maybe they also know that God will balance the scales in the end. He says, "Vengeance is mine" (Romans 12:19). No one will get away with breaking the law, unless they are forgiven in Christ. The Apostle Paul even says this, "I forget the past and strain towards what is ahead" (Philippians 3:13). Imagine if, when you drive your car, you spend the entire time looking in the rear-view mirror? What would happen? You would crash! People spend their entire life looking in the rear-view mirror of their past hurts, their past pain, their past relationships, and they crash and burn. If you want to heal, you have to learn to forgive others, so you can move forward.

Jesus realized how important forgiveness is. He not only spoke about it, he lived it! Imagine how much pain and hurt Jesus experienced, and still experiences today, yet chooses to forgive when asked. Think about all the people who still mock him, still nail him to the cross; yet, in an instant, he is ready to forgive (1 John 1:9). The Apostle Paul reminded us of this when he commanded: "Forgive others as Christ forgave you" (Ephesians 4:32). Jesus reminds us of the importance of forgiveness by including it in the prayer he taught us to pray, The Lord's Prayer: *"Forgive us our trespasses as we forgive those who trespass against us"* (Matthew 6:12). When we pray this, we are giving God permission to treat us as we treat others. If we forgive others, we will experience God's forgiveness; if we don't, we won't. This is not referring to the once-and-for-all forgiveness offered to those who accept God's love by believing in His one and only Son (John 3:16). The forgiveness that is spoken of in the Lord's Prayer is the forgiveness offered on a daily basis, which affects our relationship to God. If we don't forgive others, then we are sinning by not doing what God says to do. Unforgiveness and resentment is sin. This is why the Bible tells us to confess our sins so that we can be forgiven (1 John 1:9). When we sin, we have hindered the closeness of fellowship with God. Sin is always a barrier to our relationship with God. I know this because I am a father. Whenever my children don't do what I ask them to do, their disobedient behavior directly affects our relationship. Yes, they are still my children, but we are not close. It is the same with God, our Father. This is why it is of upmost importance to apologize to God when you sin, which includes the sin of unforgiveness, because you don't want anything to hinder the close relationship you can have with your Father in heaven.

I know what you're thinking... What about people who continue to be harmful to my family or me? Must I forgive them? The simple answer is "yes!" But let me make an important distinction. Forgiveness and trust are not one and the same. <u>Forgiveness is a gift–trust is earned</u>. Forgiveness is something you "give" someone, which is why it is called "forGIVEness." It is a gift mostly to yourself, because the other person is really never held in bondage by your unforgiveness, rather it is you who is held in bondage. So, not forgiving hinders your joy, your peace, your healing, not the other party. Trust is different than forgiveness. Trust is earned. What I mean is that in order to trust someone, there must be a history of trustworthiness. If someone is not trustworthy, then it would be foolish to trust them. You can forgive someone; yet not trust him or her. Forgiveness is a gift; trust is earned.

Forgiveness is the key to your healing. You can move through steps 1, 2, all the way to 8, but if you do not forgive, you will not heal. As I said earlier, the steps in the A, B, C's of healing only work if you work the steps. And you can't skip steps. You can't move on to step 7, "Grow," if you won't forgive.

The most important step to forgiveness is to receive God's forgiveness. Hopefully, you have done this. Hopefully you have placed your faith in God's only Son, Jesus Christ, for your eternal salvation. If you have, then your sins have all been wiped away and forgiven. All of your past sins, present sins, and future sins, are as far away from you as the east is from the west (Psalm 103:12). But the fact of the matter is, we don't live in tomorrow, we live in today. Our relationship with God is a day-to-day, minute-by-minute relationship. It is like any other relationship, I'm either growing closer to God or further apart. No relationship stays stagnant. In order for me to experience closeness with my wife, I need to admit when I'm wrong and apologize. It is the same with our Father in heaven. Whenever we realize that we have sinned, we should confess (agree) right away. Don't wait! The Apostle Paul says it this way: "Do not let the sun go down on your anger, don't give the devil a foothold" (Ephesians 4:26-27). What does he mean by this? He means that if you let sin fester, (unforgiveness is a sin), you will only be giving the Devil a foothold into areas of your life that he will try and destroy. I know of men who are deep in the throes of pornography. I know of one man who got to the point where he was having online sex with women and eventually had many affairs while married. He didn't deal with the sin in a timely manner, so the sin grew and grew until his marriage fell apart. If you don't deal with your sin, your sin will deal with you!

Jesus said, "If we confess our sins, he is faithful and just and will forgive us our sins and purify us from all unrighteousness" (1 John 1:9). Don't let the devil get a foothold in your life, your marriage, or your family. Make confession a daily discipline, and see how much better you sleep at night!

I want to close with a sobering story about a man I met a few years ago. He and his wife asked to be re-married after thirty years of being divorced. The man told me that thirty years before, he left his wife and family to do what he described as, "a stupid thing called divorce." He was too proud to apologize, and too immature to do the right thing. He went on to say, "All these years, I've lived alone, and now I see how foolish I've been. My bitterness has robbed me of the joys of life and marriage, and now I want to remarry so I can have a few of those years back." Even though his story has a happy ending, his life was filled with years of sadness and remorse due to his decision to hold on to unforgiveness, resentment, and anger. He missed God's best, because he allowed the Devil to get a foothold and not let go. Don't miss God's best. Learn the power of forgiveness.

I encourage you to pray this prayer.....

"Heavenly Father, I want to first thank you for your forgiveness. I am forever grateful for offering your forgiveness to me through your one and only Son, Jesus Christ. Now cause me to forgive others the way you have forgiven me. I don't want to hold on to resentment and anger, because I know it will only make me spiritually and physically sick. Please give me the strength to forgive those who have hurt me. Show me where there is sin in my life. When you show me, I pray that I would be faithful and quick to confess, so as to not hinder our relationship. I pray I would also repent and change my behavior. You are the most important person in my life, and I need you more than anything or

anyone else. I ask that you get rid of any pride or ego that is stopping me from being a forgiving person. When I hurt someone, I want to do the right thing by apologizing. Remind me to apologize, so that I can keep my side of the street clean. Lord Jesus, I want to be like you. You chose to forgive me even though I am undeserving. Cause me to be a forgiver like you. In Jesus' Name, Amen."

Who Do I Need To Forgive Totally?

1. _____

2. _____

3. _____

4. _____

5. _____

Step 7: *Grow*

Brothers, do not be children in your thinking. Be infants in evil, but
in your thinking be mature." – 1 Corinthians 14:20,
The Apostle Paul

a man fell in a hole. He fell in a hole, and he couldn't get out. A traveller passed by. He told the man to meditate, to purify his mind, and when he reached nirvana, all suffering would cease. The man did as he was told, but the man remained in the hole. Another man appeared. He told the man that the hole didn't exist; neither did the man. It was all an illusion. The man who did not exist was still stuck in the hole that was not there. Another visitor arrived. He instructed the man to perform good deeds, to improve his karma; and though he would still die in the hole, he might be reincarnated as something magnificent. Another man looked down from above. He taught the man to pray five times a day and follow five important tenets. One day, perhaps, the divine would set him free. The man prayed as best he could, but he started losing strength, and in the hole he remained. Another man appeared. There was something different about this man. He called down to the man in the hole and asked him if he wanted to be freed. The man answered, "yes." This man lowered himself into the hole, into the pit. He took hold of the man and dragged him into the light. And the man in the hole who could not get himself out was saved.

This story shows our plight. We, like that man, are stuck in a hole, unable to get out. We try and try our best to get ourselves out, but to no avail. That is when Jesus comes. He gets into the hole with us and pulls us out. God is the only one who can save us; he is the only one who can set us free. Once we are free, we should walk. We should take the steps assigned to us so that we can begin to grow. This is what this chapter is about – Growing.

Step 7: **Grow** in my relationship with God.

To help you grasp what it means to grow in your relationship with Christ, I have developed an acronym: G-R-O-W. I hope it will help you remember what it means to grow. This reminds me of a college professor from Yale. He was invited to speak to the student body about what it means to be a student at Yale. In order to do this, he developed an acronym built around the letters of the university: Youth, Attitude, Loyalty, and Enthusiasm. The only problem was that he spent thirty minutes on each letter. When he was finished, he walked down from the stage and asked a student in the front row, "What did you think of my lecture and my acrostic?" to which the student answered, "I'm just glad that I didn't go to the Massachusetts Institute of Technology!" Don't worry … I won't spend thirty pages on each letter. My hope is to assist you in understanding the purpose and importance of growing in your relationship with God.

G-et On The PATH

As you may know, I am the senior pastor at a church called The Gate Christian Bible Church. I am the founding pastor of this church. Serving as the pastor has been incredibly challenging, yet at the same time unbelievably rewarding. Challenges are God's ways of growing us. In fact, the Bible is filled with stories of people who were tested so that their faith would grow. Some passed with flying colors, others failed miserably. But even in failing, God was able to teach a lesson that could not be taught any other way. This is how God works. He pulls us out of the hole and then sets our feet on a PATH.

Jesus said, *"I am the gate, whoever enters through me will be saved"* (John 10:9). This means that the only way I can get to heaven is to enter through the Gate, Jesus Christ. Once I enter, through faith, I am ready to live out my faith. I do this by walking with the Lord and trusting him as he leads. In other words, I am now on a path, which consists of challenges and obstacles. I can either trust God to get me to the next place or try my own gimmicks and tricks. You know where that will get you! So, the purpose of the path is to grow your faith.

At the Gate Christian Bible Church, we also have a PATH. It stands for **P**artnership, **A**dvancement, **T**eamwork, **H**arvest. Each step on the PATH involves a commitment to God. Partnership is a commitment to Jesus Christ and to each other. Advancement is a commitment to growing. Teamwork is a commitment to serving. Harvest is a commitment to sharing your faith. Each commitment involves taking an introductory class, which explains the commitment, and offers each person the opportunity to make a commitment to walking and continuing on the PATH. The PATH is a process because our growth in Christ is also a process. We do not become

147

mature overnight. A baby doesn't become an adult when it is still a baby. It is the same with us. We do not become mature in our faith overnight; we become mature over *time*. This is important to understand. But it is also important that you do not stay as a baby; that you do not crawl back in the hole. Jesus pulled you out so you can begin to walk. So start walking.

Seeds

There's a story in the Bible about a farmer and some seeds …
Then he [Jesus] told them many things in parables, saying:
"A farmer went out to sow his seed. As he was scattering the seed,
some fell along the path, and the birds came and ate it up. Some
fell on rocky places, where it did not have much soil. It sprang up
quickly, because the soil was shallow. But when the sun came up,
the plants were scorched, and they withered because they had no
root. Other seed fell among thorns, which grew up and choked
the plants. Still other seed fell on good soil, where it produced a
crop–a hundred, sixty or thirty times what was sown.
Whoever has ears, let them hear."
- Matthew 13:3–9

Hopefully by now you have ears to hear and a heart that understands. Jesus shared this story with his disciples, and sadly they did not understand. So they did the only thing they could do, they asked Jesus to tell them what it meant. It is amazing to me how many people make decisions about Jesus and the Bible without even knowing what it means. They will reject God's Word, yet not even make a concerted effort to try and understand. The answer to what it means is right there with you – Jesus Christ! Why don't you ask him for understanding before you make a decision about what he says? At least the disciples had enough wisdom to ask for understanding.

By the way, this is a great time for me to tell you of the importance of the Church. When I say "Church", I am not speaking of a building. I am speaking of what the Bible refers to as the Body of Christ. The Church is the current expression of God's Kingdom on this earth. Jesus died for the Church; he gave his body so that we could become his body. In other words, once someone comes to faith in Christ, they are now part of his body, the Church. So think about what that means as far as you are concerned. Are you a believer? Have you placed your faith in God's one and only Son, Jesus Christ? If so, the Bible says that you are a new creation (2 Corinthians 5:17). It also says that you have died with him and are now alive with him (Romans 6). This means that you have become united with him as one. When you died to yourself and came alive in Christ, you became a part of his body, and you are now just as alive as he is. The problem is that you are currently stuck in your old body, but that won't last forever. One day, the Bible says that you will receive a new body, a body just like Jesus' body. But for now, you are a new person stuck in an old body. So why didn't God take you to heaven the moment you believed? I mean, wouldn't that be better? Imagine the freedom and peace you would experience in heaven where there is no more death, no more pain, and no more sickness. Why did God leave you here? He left you here so you can grow. And the way you grow is to be an active participant in his Body, the Church. If you are not an active member of a local Church, you will never become who you are intended to be. Your growth will be stunted. Get plugged into a local church that teaches the Bible. I promise, you will begin to grow because growth happens within the Body.

Now back to the story of the seeds. Jesus says that the farmer scattered some seed along the path. The path is where the seed is scattered, and the seed is the Word of God, as the disciples found out later after asking Jesus what this story meant. What happened to the seed that fell on the path? The birds came up and ate it. Now think about this... Are these birds, good birds or bad birds?

I remember the old Alfred Hitchcock movie, "The Birds". That movie was scary because the birds outnumbered the people. They came in droves and drove the people out of their town. They were evil birds. The birds in this story are also evil. How do I know this? They are evil because they stole the seed from the path. The seed is the Word of God, and these evil birds took the seed from the ground. It is important to note that the different ground described in this story describes the condition of the soil. The soil represents your heart. Once the Word of God is spoken, the seed falls on to the soil (the human heart). According to this story, some seed is taken away, some is rejected, and some falls on good fertile soil. In the first description, the seed falls on the path, and the evil birds take it away. These birds represent the evil one – your Adversary – the Devil. He never wants anyone to receive God's Word. He knows the power of God's spoken Word and will do whatever he can to try and take it away. This is why it is SO important that the moment you place your faith in Christ is the moment you need to start to grow. If you don't, the seed might be taken away. This is the first soil – the heart that doesn't do its part to grow by getting involved with the Body. This seed is taken away.

The second soil is referred to as "rocky". Have you ever tried to plant seeds in rocky soil? We live in an area of Orange County where the soil is rather hard. The other day, we were digging down into the soil, and in a matter of a few inches we hit rock. We were wondering why anything we planted in that soil would not grow. The reason nothing grew was due to the condition of the soil. The rocky soil represents a heart that receives the seed (the Word of God) but because their heart is not pliable, the seed cannot take root. When the troubles of the world come upon them, because they have no root, they quickly fall away. This is all due to the condition of the heart. This person, rather than letting the *Word* take root, they let the *world* take root, and they reject the seed rather than receive it.

The third soil is described as "thorny soil". The person who has this kind of heart is more interested in "thorny" things such as wealth and worry than growth in God's Word. I have this unusual interest in tumbleweeds. When I was young, I would hope to see tumbleweeds. Something about tumbleweeds peeked my curiosity – where did they come from, why are they round, how do they keep their shape? Tumbleweed is a fragment of a plant. Once this fragment becomes dry, it detaches from the rest of the plant and its root, and tumbles away in the wind. This is such a picture of many people in our world today. These people heard the Word of God preached, they might have even gone to church on a regular basis, but because they are not receiving the Word into their heart, they become dry; they start to detach from their root – Jesus Christ – and the rest of the plant – the Church – and get blown away by the winds of this world.

The fourth soil is the good, fertile soil. This is someone who hears the Word and understands it. This person receives God's Word into their heart because they have received The Word, Jesus Christ. They hunger and thirst for the Word of God because they realize it gives life to their parched soul. You can spot this person in a crowd because the seed has taken root; therefore, they produce a lot of fruit, a huge crop. God uses these types of people in mighty ways, and the Church and the world notices.

Which type of person are you? How fertile is your heart? Growing people get on the path and stay on the path. They walk with God and are active members in his church. They produce a lot of fruit, which causes the church to grow and be healthy. These people become spiritually mature. This is the type of person I pray you become.

R-ely on God's Grace

The man in the hole had a huge problem. He could not get out of the hole by his own strength. God had to come and pull him out. This is grace. The Bible says that we are saved by grace, not by works (Ephesians 2:8). This means that there is nothing you could ever do to earn your way to heaven. The only person who can get you to heaven is the person who pulled you out of the hole, Jesus Christ, God's Son. Grace is undeserved favor. God, in his compassion and grace, sent his Son to pull you out of the hole. You didn't deserve it, yet you accept it, because you realize that without God's grace, you would still be in that hole. But grace is even more than just an act of love and compassion. Grace is a source of power. Dallas Willard says this about grace: "The true saint burns grace like a 747 burns fuel on takeoff." Grace doesn't just pull us out of the hole; grace keeps us from going into the hole again! When I rely on grace, I can stay out of the hole. On the other hand, when I rely on my own strength, I will inevitably end up back in the hole. This is what happened to me when I ended up in rehab. I tried to solve my problems on my own and ended up back in the hole. But because of God's grace, he pulled me out yet again! Even though that experience was very painful, he still used that horrible time of my life in a powerful way. He taught me so many things, and the evidence is in the words of this book! God never wastes a hurt, and he always turns what is bad into good if we trust him.

He Holds Your Hand

In Phoenix, Arizona, a 26-year-old mother stared down at her son who was dying of terminal leukemia. Her heart was filled with sadness, but also a strong feeling of determination. She took her son's hand and asked, "Billy, did you ever think about what you wanted to be when you grew up?"

"Mommy, I always wanted to be a fireman." His Mom smiled back and said, "Let's see if we can make your dream come true."

Later that day, she talked to Fireman Bob. She asked if it might be possible for her 6-year-old son to ride around the block on a fire engine. He said, "We can do better than that.

Have your son ready at 7:00a.m. Wednesday morning. We're going to make him an honorary fireman the whole day. We'll give him his own fire suit and everything."

Wednesday morning came, and Fireman Bob picked up Billy, dressed him in his fire suit, and escorted him from his hospital bed to the waiting hook and ladder truck. There were three fire calls in Phoenix that day, and Billy got to go on all the calls. He was in heaven! With all the love that was lavished on him, Billy lived three months longer than anticipated. But, one night, things fell for the worse. His vital signs dropped, and the nurse called the family members to the hospital. Fireman Bob found out, and in honor of little Billy, he sent the hook and ladder truck with sirens blaring to Billy's hospital window. He told everyone that the fire department was going to visit one of their finest members one last time. Sixteen firefighters climbed the latter to Billy's third floor window and entered his room. Billy was impressed. He looked up and asked, "Chief, am I really a fireman now?" "Yes, Billy, you are, and the Head Chief, Jesus, is holding your hand." With those words, Billy smiled and said, "I know, He's been holding my hand all day, and the angels have been singing." He closed his eyes one last time.

God is the one who holds your hand and brings you home. This is only by his grace. Without his grace, we would be hopeless, but because of his grace, we remain hopeful. We remain hopeful even when things aren't going the way we would like. We realize that God is holding our hand even when we feel alone. God has strong hands; he not only pulls us out of the pit, he walks with us on the path. We can rely on God's faithfulness because he always keeps his promise. He has promised to finish what he started in you (Philippians 1:6). You can count on God to be there no matter what!

White-Knuckling It

Before we move on to the next topic, I must spend a little time talking about something known as "white-knuckling it". The words, "white-knuckle" are often used to describe a scary situation, i.e. a roller coaster; the person holds on so hard that his knuckles turn white. In terms of healing, to white-knuckle means to hold on instead of let go. The person with the destructive behavior may stop performing the behavior, but is not living a life of solution; he lives a life of confusion. Instead of relying on God's grace, the one who white-knuckles, tries to power himself into a solution, rather than relying on God's grace and power as the solution. People like this may last a long time, they may seem happy and content, but deep down they are still very unhappy and anxious. I lived like this for a long time. Even though I stopped the destructive behavior, I was unhappy because I tried to solve my problem in my own strength. This would lead to outbursts of anger, treating those whom I love the most the worst, because I would try and hide my problems so that others would not see. I was wearing a mask; I was not honest. Therefore, I was losing the battle, and eventually my problem got the best of me because I could not hang on any longer. My advice to you is to NOT try and white-knuckle your way out of a problem. Instead, I encourage you to rely on God's grace and the help of others, so that you will be truly healed. Don't try so hard to hold on, let God hold on to you.

O-bey God's Commands

The evening before Jesus was crucified for our sins, he said a lot of important things about God's plan and his will for those who would follow him. He spoke of a "helper" who would come and give us power to live the Christian life. This "helper" we know as the Holy Spirit. The Holy Spirit would come and dwell in the hearts of those who called Jesus their Lord. The Holy Spirit is the one who gives us the strength and grace to live according to God's plan. The problem though is that even though we may have the Spirit, often times the Spirit does not have us. In other words, we do not submit to the Holy Spirit's leadership in our lives. This means that we live in disobedience to God's plan. This causes all kinds of problems that cause us to deter from God's path. God's Spirit and His Word work together in tandem. When someone who has the Spirit does not live according to His Word, he or she will experience more problems than if they would submit to God's authority. This is not only evident in the lives of those who disobey, it was also predicted by Jesus. While he was in the room with his disciples the night before he died, he said this: "If you love me, you will obey my commands" (John 14:15).

I love my wife very much. She is God's gift to me. But what if I never told her I loved her? What would that do with regards to our relationship? Some might say, "My wife knows I love her", and that is fine if you were not in relation with her. But relationships demand attention. This attention often comes through communication. If I'm not willing to communicate my love to my wife, do I really love her? And if I really do love her, it is imperative that I tell her and show her. Well, guess what? You are in a relationship with God. All relationships demand respect for the other. When Jesus tells us that if we love him, we will do what he says, what does that mean? It means this: When I don't do what God says, I am not loving him. I have heard people verbally communicate their love for God, yet their actions prove otherwise. How can someone love God when they won't do what he says? What kind of love is that? That, my friends, is love for self, not for God. When I love myself, my desires, and my objectives, more than I love God, it will appear in my decisions and my actions. I will make decisions according to my will, rather than God's will. I will travel away from God's path and forge a path of my own. You have to realize something ... if you want more problems than you already have, then continue to love yourself more than you love God. Continue to think that you know all the answers instead of trusting God for the answers. I speak from experience, not only in my own life, but also in those whom I pastor. I have seen well-intentioned Christians turn their back on God's commands and end up in terrible situations. As I've said before, good intentions are not enough. We need good direction. Good direction comes from our Good Shepherd, Jesus Christ.

There are many stories in the Bible of people who lost their way because they rejected God's directions. One person in particular was very important. You have probably heard of him because he is one of the most well known people to ever live. His name is Moses, and he was the leader God used to release the Israelites from Egyptian slavery. God referred to Moses as his friend, and also referred to him as the most humble man to ever live. But Moses also had a problem, an anger problem, as displayed one time when Moses, in anger, murdered another man. This person, Moses, is the person God used so tremendously! I don't know about you, but this gives me hope!

Striking The Rock

As much as Moses was a godly man, he was also an angry man. After God miraculously delivered his people out of Egypt by way of the Red Sea, he led them on an excursion through the desert. His intent was that they would move into their new land quickly, but because of Israel's unbelief, they spent a generation (40 years) on a long walk. God had to teach them a lesson. By the way, this is also a lesson to us. When we don't trust God, we will have to go around the desert a few times until we learn what he is trying to teach us. My prayer is always, "Lord, whatever you're desiring to teach me, cause me to learn it quickly!" I don't want to live my life wandering around the desert; I want to enter the Promised Land!

Moses was a leader of trepidation. He did not want to lead these, as God called them, "stiff-necked" people. But Moses also knew that this was his destiny. Everything was going well until Moses lost his temper one day. The people started complaining to Moses about the lack of food and water. So God sent bread from heaven, and water from a rock. God told Moses to strike the rock and water would gush forth. We find out later that this rock was the spiritual manifestation of God's Son, Jesus Christ. This makes perfect sense since it was Jesus who stood in Jerusalem saying loudly, "If anyone is thirsty, come to me and drink" (John 7:37). As the Jews marched around that desert, they got thirsty again. They started complaining and nagging Moses for more water. God told Moses to *speak* to the rock. But, in anger, Moses *struck* the rock. Now, you would think that this would be a minor offense. I mean, speak and strike both start with the same letter. Plus, God had told him before to strike the rock, so Moses may have just misunderstood. But what happened to Moses almost doesn't seem fair. Because Moses struck the rock instead of speaking, he missed out on entering the Promised Land! What? Yes, you heard me correctly. Moses, God's friend, the most famous man in the Bible, made a costly mistake, which to us seems minor, and this mistake kept him out of experiencing God's promise.

Now, before we go on, you must understand that the mistake did not keep him out of heaven; for it was Moses, along with Elijah, who fellowshipped with Jesus Christ on the Mount of Transfiguration. But Moses was left out of enjoying the land of Canaan here on earth. He died in the desert along with all the other grumblers and sinners. Why do you think God took Moses' mistake so seriously? The answer lies in what Moses said just before, and what God said just after the rock-striking event. In anger, Moses said this: "Listen, you rebels, must <u>we</u> bring you water out of this rock?" (Numbers 20:10). I underlined the word "we" because that is an important word. The question goes back to who provided the water from the rock. Was it Moses or God? It was God. But Moses said, "we". This is the problem when we try and impose ourselves into the place where God alone reigns. We do this all the time. Instead of giving credit where credit is due, we take the credit. It's all about me and we instead of He and Him! But even at this, you would think, is that enough to cause God's friend to die in the desert? What God said after this event is the main reason Moses died with the rest. "But the Lord said to Moses and Aaron, 'Because you did not trust in me enough to honor me as holy in the sight of the Israelites, you will not bring this community into the land I give them" (Numbers 20:12). What was the main reason Moses was left out? He did not TRUST God. Moses white-knuckled it. In his anger, he pushed God away. He did not trust God enough to do what he said. Sure, it was just a mistake, but it was a huge mistake. It wasn't as if Moses didn't know God's commands. It was Moses to whom God gave the Ten Commandments! They spent days on the mountain together talking. If there was anyone who knew God's voice, it was Moses. Yet, Moses didn't listen. He didn't trust God. Instead, he took the reins and tried to do things his way. Moses did not obey God's commands.

Now, how do you fit into this narrative? If you are a believer in Jesus Christ, then you, like Moses, know God very well. The reason you know God very well is because you know Jesus, and he knows you. The Seed has been planted in your heart. God speaks to you on a regular basis; you know his voice. In fact, Jesus said that those who follow him would know his voice. Yet, like Moses, you push God away. Whether it is through unresolved anger, unforgiveness, pride, or any other sin, we tend to miss what God says, because our ears are only in tune with our desires, rather than God's. The difference between you and Moses, however, is that Moses lived during a time when God dealt with his people a little differently. Israel, like the Church, was called to be different, but the difference is that Israel is a nation of people, whereas the Church is a community of people. The reason we know this is because God had a certain land chosen for Israel, whereas our land is in heaven. God was forming Israel into a nation that would rule the world, and Moses was her leader. But God was the true leader of Israel. Israel was meant to be a theocracy. When Moses usurped God's leadership, he usurped the purpose of Israel – to be a people under the authority of God. If God could not be Israel's leader, then Israel would be just like every other nation on the face of this earth, and that was not God's intent.

Even though the Church is not Israel, nevertheless we act like Israel all the time. We grumble, we complain, we stop trusting and obeying; we usurp God's leadership. Instead of our life being a Theocracy, we live in a democracy. Democracy might be great for our nation, but it is not great for your relationship with God. He has to be in charge; otherwise, he will have to do what he did to Israel. Why? ...Because, he loves you. He does not want you to love any-thing or anyone more than him. He knows that if you do, your growth will be stunted. But thank God for his grace that we won't die in the desert! Because of Jesus Christ, we will live eternally with God. But this does not mean we won't suffer consequences for our sinful behavior. When we strike the rock instead of speak to the rock, as God instructs, we are saying to God, "I don't trust you; I know what is best for me you don't!" This is our plight, and this is what shows our sinful nature. Disobeying God's commands is dangerous, dan-gerous enough to cause you to miss God's best.

<u>W</u>-orship Him Only

Some of the things that are hard for people to understand have to do with what we call "Christian-ese" terms. These are words that are indigenous to the Church community and sometimes do not make sense to others, especially to those who are not on the path or just entering the path. One of these words is the word, "worship." Although we worship things and people all the time, we don't know what the term means with regards to the Bible. To worship means to love or adore: to express your love for someone or something. The very first commandment God gave his people was this: "Thou shalt not have any other gods above me" (Deuteronomy 5:7). God loves his people so much that he knew that if they loved other things (we might call them idols) more than him, these things would not satisfy, they would only disappoint and cause hurt and pain. The reason God gives commands is for the protection of those he loves. When we love things or people more than God, we are opening the door to pain and disappointment. When we love God more than anything else, we will open the door to health, well-being, and success. So to worship God only means to love him more than anyone or anything else.

I used to love music and fame more than God. I used to live to make a name of myself. This was idolatry at its core, because those things (music and fame) will not satisfy the hunger and thirst I have for God. Sure, those things might satisfy for a moment, but eventually you will either have to have more or you will move on to something else. This was the problem with the pills the doctor gave me. At first they satisfied and actually made me feel more like myself. But after a while, the dosage was not meeting the need, so I had to up the dosage. This type of behavior will continue until I realize I need help or something worse happens. When someone loves God more than anything or anyone else, he will be satisfied, not just for a moment, but for eternity.

Expensive Perfume

Just this week I heard of a person who found some old baseball cards in a plastic bag, and the cards are worth one million dollars! Imagine finding something this costly. What would you do? There was a woman who had saved up enough money to buy a bottle of expensive perfume. She might have even planned on using it on her wedding night. This perfume was very valuable to this woman. What she did instead is a story for the ages. It is found in the Bible in John chapter twelve. Jesus was invited over to the house of a very important man. While Jesus was getting ready to eat, a woman came in. She is described as a very sinful woman. Many believe she used to live a life of ill-repute, maybe even a prostitute. But this woman heard about Jesus. She entered the room and opened her expensive bottle of perfume; she began to wash Jesus' feet with it. As she washed his feet, she began to kiss his feet and wipe them with her hair. The men in the room were astonished and quickly came to judgment saying, "if this man [Jesus] were truly a prophet, he would know who this woman was" (Luke 7:39). Jesus did know who she was, but he did not stop her from doing what she came to do. You see, this woman came to worship Jesus. She didn't care what it cost, because she loved him that much. This is what true worship is – expressing your love to God. When someone loves someone else, they stop at nothing to show their love.

When my wife and I started dating, I would want to spend every minute of every day with her. I would buy her gifts and treat her as if she were worth more than gold. Over time, sadly, our desire to spend time together diminished. This was due mostly to the cares of the world, and also trying to raise three children. This is the case with many marriages and relationships. We get busy and our relationships suffer. This is also the case with Jesus. We start out loving him with a passionate heart, wanting to spend time with him, holding back nothing, not even our expensive perfume. But over time, we get too busy for Jesus, and our relationship suffers. This world is full of distractions; it will cause you to neglect your relationships, especially your most important ones. Our relationship with God is the most important relationship we will ever have. In other parts of the world, people stay focused much better, because they are not as distracted as we are. Jesus is all they have. Here's the bottom line: Jesus won't be all you want until you realize Jesus is all you have. When you realize this, you will hold back nothing. You will open up your expense account and wash his feet with it. This is true worship – giving everything you have to Jesus. This starts with giving your life, and then everything else will follow.

Now, it's interesting to see the response from the others in the room when this woman poured out her perfume. The man who invited Jesus was astonished. Jesus answered by telling a story of two people who owed money to a lender. One owed a lot, and one owed a little. The lender decided to forgive their debt. Jesus asked, "who do you think was more grateful?" "The one who had the bigger debt forgiven," the man answered (Luke 7:43). The point here is that this woman who poured her expensive perfume over Jesus' feet knew how much she owed Jesus for forgiving her. Worship is an outflow of a person's heart. When someone realizes just how much Jesus did for him or her, that person will hold nothing back. They will realize the amount of forgiveness they have received from Jesus, and they too, will pour out their worship, their love and adoration, upon Jesus.

The other person who responded was Judas Iscariot. Judas was one of Jesus' disciples, but he was the one who would eventually betray Jesus for a few coins. Judas was also in charge of the money. He was Jesus' treasurer who would often steal from the treasury account. Judas became extremely upset that this woman would "waste" this expensive perfume on Jesus. First of all, the word "waste" is a subjective term found only in the eye of the beholder. The woman did not think she was wasting anything. In fact, she probably felt like she was doing what any person should do, when they realize the depth of God's love offered through His Son, Jesus Christ. But because Judas was distracted by the things of the world, and he was only focused on himself, he thought it better to take the perfume and sell it. He wanted to put the money in the treasury account so he would have more to steal from. There are many people like this. They don't want to express their love for Jesus because they are only interested in what they can get out of it, not what they can give to God and to others. This attitude is called stinginess. You will never heal if you are stingy. You will only become more bitter and resentful. Express your love to God. Open up your bottle of expensive perfume, and pour it out. When you do this, I can promise you this: Not only will you show just how much you love Jesus, you will also cause the world to smell a whole lot better!

A Barren Womb

King David was the second king of Israel. Saul, the first king, blew it big time. Therefore, God turned the kingdom over to David, a man after God's own heart. David was an Old Testament man living in a New Testament world. What I mean is that David understood the grace and forgiveness of God. You can read about it in the Psalms, as David wrote many of them. David was a fighter, a warrior. He won many battles for Israel. One battle won caused him to return the Ark of the Covenant back to Israel. The Ark was very important to Israel, as it housed the Ten Commandments along with other important artifacts of God's faithfulness. The Philistines had stolen the ark, and Israel had to get it back. David, filled with joy, danced in the streets because of the victory that was won. But his wife looked out the window at David, and the Bible says she despised him in her heart (2 Samuel 6:16). Why would David's wife despise him just for dancing with joy?

There are people who are not happy when someone worships God. They have a hard heart and hate it when God is worshipped. These types of people look out their window judging those who love God. They mock them and despise them in their heart. David's wife paid the consequences for despising her husband. The Bible says that she was not able to have children (2 Samuel 6:23). When someone refuses to worship God, they become barren. Worship unleashes God's power and presence. When someone refuses to worship, he or she will not experience the power and presence of God and, therefore, remain spiritually barren. If you want to be healed and experience life in all its fullness, then worship God!

Your Spiritual Tool Box

When you were born, you entered this world with an empty toolbox. Then over time, you started to fill your toolbox with tools that work and tools that don't work. Depending on your circumstances and experiences, you either learned how to handle life's struggles in a healthy way or an unhealthy way. The tools you use to handle life's challenges are based on which tools you used in the past. If I want to tighten a bolt I should not use a hammer, I should use a wrench. If I want to drill a hole, I shouldn't use an axe. When I enter into conflict, the way I handle the conflict depends on which tools I pull out of my spiritual and emotional toolbox. For me, I learned that expressing my feelings was wrong, and if I did express them, no one listened. I felt invalidated. Therefore, I learned that conflict was never good, because it would end up with me being taken advantage of. The other party would not listen nor care. This caused me to fight to get a word in edgewise instead of learning the important art of listening. The tools I grab to handle conflict are not the right tools at all. The only way that I can replace the tools I used in the past with new tools, is to unlearn what I previously learned, and learn a new way to deal with life. This is called "repentance". I repent when I stop believing what I used to believe was true, and start believing in what God says is true. The first act of repentance in someone's life is to believe in Jesus Christ. From that point on, God is going to fill your toolbox with new tools. He does this by his Word and through his Spirit, and by your repentance. God cannot force you to repent; this has to be a choice you make on your own. When you repent you will see God's power and grace working in your life like he intended. This is how you grow, by repenting and trusting God to give you the right tools to live an abundant life. This is why growing in your relationship with God is so important.

Imagine if you paid hundreds of dollars to take piano lessons but never practiced. I meet people like this all the time. They want to have all the benefit without any of the work. This will get you nowhere.

Achieving something takes hard work. Imagine if you spent thousands of dollars on a college education but never showed up for class. This would be stupid to say the least. People do this all the time with God. God has paid an incredible price for you. He gave his Son to die on your behalf. Yet many people don't realize what they have received and just go about life the same way they used to live. They don't show up to church, they don't serve God or others. They find themselves back in a hole because they never did their part. Growing takes work. My children are grown now and they are going out on their own. They could not do the things they are doing now as children. They had to grow up. Don't stay as a child in your relationship with God. Grow! Put in the work. Show up and suit up. No one can grow for you. You have to want to grow and you have to want to change.

The Bible exhorts me not to conform to the ways of this world, but rather to be transformed by the renewing of my mind (Romans 12:2). The only way that my mind can be renewed is by the Word of God. I have to un-learn what I learned before, and learn what God wants me to know now. He wants me to know about His Son, about his plan for my life, and about the new tools that come in my new toolbox. Here are some of the things you should start to do so that God can fill your toolbox with His Word:

1) You need to be saved. You can only become new by God's Spirit, and the only way you receive God's Spirit is through faith in God's Son, Jesus Christ. This means you must enter the Gate of salvation. That is your first step to growing and to gaining new tools.

2) Get on the PATH. Find a local church where you can grow in your relationship with God and His Body, the Church.

Become a *Partner* with others in growing, *Advance* beyond where you are to where God is taking you, *Team* up with others so you can learn and grow together, and start sharing your faith with others because as Jesus said, "The *Harvest* is plenty, but the workers are few" (Matthew 9:37).

3) Start a healing process. There are so many good programs to help you heal and recover from your past hurts, habits, and hang-ups. Celebrate Recovery is a Christian-based recovery program that is implemented all over the world (celebraterecovery.com). Or start a new *Healing Steps* program in your church. We can help train you and provide everything you need to get started. Visit *thegatecbc.com* for more information.

When you start implementing these growth steps into your life, you will start to heal, and you will begin to gather healthy tools to deal with the struggles and problems of life. It won't happen overnight, so make sure you stay on the path. Don't give up, because remember, your miracle may be just around the corner.

Step 8: *Help*

"The King will reply, 'Truly I tell you, whatever you did for one of the least of these brothers and sisters of mine, you did for me."
– Matthew 25:40, Jesus Christ

"He comforts us in all our troubles so that we can comfort others. When they are troubled, we will be able to give them the same comfort God has given us."– 2 Corinthians 1:4, *The Apostle Paul*

 ith two runners on base and a strike against her, Sara Tucholsky of Western Oregon University uncorked her best swing ever and did something she had never done before in high school or college–she hit a home run. Her first home run of her career cleared the centerfield fence. But it appeared to be the shortest of dreams come true when she missed first base, started back to tag it, and collapsed with a knee injury. She crawled back to first base, but could do no more. Her teammates ran out to help, but were stopped by the first-base coach. He knew that if they helped their teammate, the entire team would be disqualified. The umpire offered a solution, saying that a pinch runner could be called in, but the homer would only count as a single. In order for the homerun to count, Sara had to make it around all the bases and touch home base, but that was not going to happen outside of a miracle. Then, something happened that changed the entire atmosphere. The members of the Central Washington University softball team, Sara's opponents, came out from their dugout and stood at first base. Two of the players decided to help. They picked Sara up and started to carry her. The spectators were stunned as the opposing team carried Sara around the bases, touching her leg to each base as they passed by. This act would eliminate them from the playoffs, yet they chose to do it anyway. As Sara was carried around the bases, the crowd cheered, and when they touched home base, the entire Oregon team was in tears. After the game, Oregon's coach was quoted as saying, "In the end, it is not about winning and losing so much as it was about this girl. She hit the ball over the fence and was in pain, and she deserved a home run." But this would have never happened if not for the help that came by way of the opposing team.

It's not enough to heal; you must help others heal. This is the eighth step on the road to the A, B, C's of healing:

Step 8: **Help** others heal

Healing Steps, the A, B, C's of healing, is a process of healing. It can help you realize that your problems can be solved, if you allow God to solve them his way, in his time. But if that were it – if it were only about you – then what is it worth? There are many people who can't run the bases; they are injured and stuck. They don't know of a way out, yet they deserve a homerun. You are the person who can help them heal by carrying them around the bases; by helping them find the path to healing. *"He comforts us in all our troubles so that we can comfort others. When they are troubled, we will be able to give them the same comfort God has given us"* (2 Corinthians 1:4). God has healed you, not so you can just experience a better life, but so that you can help someone else find life. It is your duty to bring someone along on the healing steps, so they can come to the same realization to what you have come: God is the one who is able to solve your problems.

When you get on an airplane, while you taxi to the runway, the flight attendants train you in case of an emergency. During your training you are told that in case of losing air pressure, an oxygen mask will drop down in front of you. What are you to do with that mask? If you are alone, then you can just put it on your own face, but if you are travelling with someone who is more vulnerable, a child, someone who is not able to help themselves, then it is your responsibility to first put a mask on that person and then put it on yourself. Why is this important? It is important because the people who cannot put on their own mask need help. There are many people in your airplane (your life) who are not able to attend to their own mask. They are hurting, in pain, experiencing the problems of life, and need your help. It is your responsibility to offer help to them.

When I was young, I wanted to be a doctor. In fact I attended college as a pre-med student; but I quickly realized that chemistry would be my downfall, so I switched to music. Having the desire to help people by being a doctor was not enough. I lacked the ability to excel in chemistry. The reason I lacked this ability was because I was not trained properly. I didn't have the proper tools in my toolbox. You now have the proper tools to help others heal. You now have the ability to help others, and this is your assignment.

Throughout this book we have looked at people in the Bible who experienced problems. You might think that you are not like them. You might think that you cannot help others because you are barely helping yourself. If you think this, then you have missed the entire point of this book. We cannot help ourselves; this is exactly why we need God. But you can help God help others. What I mean is that God has left you here for a purpose. Why didn't he just snatch you up to heaven when you were saved? I mean, wouldn't that have been better? He left you here for a reason. Now, think about this for a moment... There are only two things you cannot do in heaven: 1) Sin; 2) Help others believe and heal. Now which do you think God left you here to do? He did not leave you here to sin; he left you here to help others heal by believing in Jesus Christ! And by the way, if you think the people in the Bible are any different than you, think of this:

Abraham was old
Jacob was insecure
Leah was unattractive
Joseph was abused
Moses stuttered
Gideon was poor
Samson was codependent
Rahab was immoral
David had an affair and all kinds of family problems
Elijah was suicidal
Jeremiah was depressed
Jonah was reluctant
Naomi was a widow
John the Baptist was eccentric, to say the least
Peter was impulsive and hot-tempered
Martha worried a lot

The Samaritan Woman had several failed marriages
Zacchaeus was unpopular
Thomas had doubts
Paul had poor health
Timothy was timid

There really is no excuse for not helping others heal.

It is interesting that one of the first things someone will ask you to do when you start attending a 12-step meeting is show up early to make coffee. Why do they do this? They do this to instill in the person that it is no longer about them. In fact, if you want to heal, it cannot be about you; it has to be about God and about others. The New Testament is filled with the following two words: "One Another." In fact, over thirty times God instructs those who are in the Church to do something good for another: "Love one another," "Welcome one another," "Accept one another," "Pray for one another," "Help one another." Why does God go out of his way to tell us this? Because he knows that when we can turn our eyes away from ourselves to helping someone else, we will not only help others heal, but <u>we</u> will also heal.

Maybe you have heard the saying, "Those who teach, can't." In other words, they are saying that if you are a music teacher or a math teacher or any kind of teacher, you are teaching because you did not have what it takes to succeed as a professional musician, or scientist. That is not true. The reason people teach, or at least it should be the reason, is to help others learn what you have learned. But it doesn't end there. Yes, the teacher helps others learn, but at the same time they are learning themselves. Helping someone learn music helps the teacher learn as well. When I teach a Bible lesson, I am not just helping someone learn, I am learning along with him or her. When I help someone heal, I too heal. This is the miracle that comes along with teaching and helping. If you truly want to experience a deep eternal healing, then help others heal.

You may not know who Natalie Gilbert is. She is a singer who was asked to sing the Star Spangled Banner for a 2003 basketball playoff game between the Portland Trailblazers and the Dallas Mavericks. Being asked to sing the National Anthem at a sporting event is a great honor, especially for Natalie who was just thirteen years old at the time. Natalie started out great. The TV camera was right in her face for the entire world to see. Then, Natalie did something that every singer fears. She forgot the words! Right in the middle of the song, she had to stop and start over, not just once, but twice! How embarrassing! Can you imagine how she must have felt? She was all by herself, out there with no one to help. That was what she thought. But the reality for Natalie was that she was not alone, there was someone sitting on the sideline that was ready to help. His name is Maurice Cheeks. He was the head coach for the Portland Trailblazers. I'm not sure what prompted Cheeks to do this, but as Natalie struggled for the entire world to see, Maurice entered the TV picture like a well-trained singing coach. The problem was that Maurice Cheeks could not carry a tune in a bucket. But he didn't care. He saw someone who was struggling, someone who needed help. So, with a loud out-of-tune voice, he put his arm around Natalie and sang with her. He helped her find her place. She got back on track and nailed it! The audience went wild!

This is a picture of what happens when we help someone get back on track. We may feel unqualified, but it doesn't matter. What matters is that someone cares enough to help. Someone comes along and puts his or her arms around you and helps you sing. Natalie Gilbert was able to finish the song because someone stood next to her with his arm around her and encouraged her to finish. He did something that she will never forget. When you help someone, you will do something they will never forget; you will help them finish. This is what Jesus Christ did for you. He came along at just the right time, put his arms around you, and helped you sing. Jesus Christ gave up his oxygen mask and gave it to you. We are to do the same.

One night a small little voice was heard from the bedroom across the hall. "Daddy, I'm scared!" The response came quick: "Honey, don't be afraid, daddy's right across the hall." After a very brief pause, the little voice is heard again, "I'm still scared!" Again a response: "You don't need to be afraid. God is watching over you." This time the pause is longer ... but the voice returns, "Daddy, I want someone with skin on!" You are Jesus with skin on. You are someone who can help someone who is scared. We are the ones that will help others heal!

How do you help others heal? This is the subject matter of the next section. But remember, this is not an exhaustive list. You will have to experiment by trying out some tools from your toolbox. God made you a certain way, with a certain personality, with certain gifts, abilities and talents. There is no one else like you. So you will be able to reach someone whom I might not be able to reach. This is the great thing about God. He knows exactly what someone needs, exactly when he or she might need it. That is your job – to find out what they need and then help provide it. Here are some things everyone can do to help others heal.

Pray for Them

I hope you have discovered the power of prayer by now. I hope that you are praying and communicating with God on a regular basis. Make sure to tap into his power, not just your own power. Jesus encouraged us to pray for our "daily bread." Praying for our own need is important, but if you really want to experience the power of prayer, start praying for others! I have had the opportunity to see God work in such powerful ways as I have prayed for the needs of others. One such person had stage 4-colon cancer. He was told that he would only live a few months. This man lived for almost 6 years! I credit this obviously to the grace of God, and also the prayer of those who prayed continually for his healing. I also shared how God touched my dad's leg and healed it while we were praying. I have seen big prayers answered and also "small" prayers. I have seen my son pray for which baseball team to sign up for. I have watched as my wife prayed to find her lost wallet and see it show up a few days later. I have prayed for protection over my children and see how God protects them even when the car accident should have caused much more serious damage. I can see God work in the big things and the small things. This causes me to be grateful, which is one of the keys to experiencing the full healing of God. I am not always grateful, but when I remember all that God has done, I become more grateful. This is why prayer is so important. Prayer helps someone be a part of what God is doing on this earth. Being a part of what God is doing is incredibly fulfilling. You can experience this fulfillment by praying for others and seeing God work in their lives.

Prayer is just communicating with God. It is talking and listening to God. Just this morning God answered a prayer. I have been looking, for all things, an accordion. Yes, I have to admit I am a recovering accordion player! But the accordion I have is not working correctly and is too big. I have been looking online but an accordion is like a guitar, you have to try it out before you buy it. This morning I prayed, "Lord, please lead me to where you want me to get an accordion." As I was leaving the gym, a lady whom I met a few weeks earlier, called my name and told me that she had heard one of my songs online and really liked it. She then told me that her husband had played trumpet at a church I used to attend. I then asked her if she played an instrument. She answered by telling me that no one wants her to play in the band. "Why?" I asked. She told me it is because she plays the accordion. "What?" I could not believe my ears. I had just prayed for God to lead me to where to get an accordion and this lady in the gym, whom I just recently met, plays accordion. Not only that, she wants to sell one of her accordions! Not only that, her accordion is the smaller compact size! Today I prayed, and today God answered! And I got it for a very reasonable price. What can I say, but that God cares about everything, even accordions! But the key to the answer was in the "ask." I had to ask. It is not that God doesn't already know what I need; it is that when I ask, I give God the opportunity to answer my request in a way that shows he cares. If I don't ask, then I won't notice the answer. Have you asked God in prayer lately? Ask and see what happens!

The Real Lord's Prayer

You can pray by even just reading the Bible. When you read the Bible, you are praying because you are communicating with God on a one-on-one basis. There are so many prayers written on the pages of the Bible. You can learn so much by reading the prayers of those who have come before us. The greatest prayer is the Lord's Prayer. I'm not speaking of the prayer we have come to know as the "Lord's Prayer." I am speaking of the actual *Lord's Prayer*. This prayer is found in John chapter seventeen. Jesus, the night before he was crucified for our sins, prayed a prayer. He prayed for his disciples who were with him then, and he also prayed for those who would be his disciples later. In essence, he prayed for you and for me! We can learn a lot about how to pray for others by studying his prayer.

Jesus' prayer is found in John chapter 17, verses 1-26. The first thing we will notice about Jesus' prayer is that "he looked toward heaven and prayed" (17:1). It is important to remember where your help comes from. Psalm 121 tells us "my help comes from the Lord" (121:2). Jesus, although being God, put aside his privileges and approached his father in heaven with humility. When Jesus starts his prayer, he says, "Father, the hour has come" (John 17:1). Notice that he refers to God as his Father. He tells us that we can approach God as our Father. A father is someone who cares. God cares about his children. We become his children when we trust his Son. In verse 6 of John 17, Jesus switches from speaking to his Father about his relationship with him to speaking to his Father about those he loves.

In his prayer, he asks his Father specific things regarding his disciples. He asks first for protection: *"Holy Father, protect them by the power of your name, the name you gave me, so that they may be one as we are one. While I was with them, I protected them and kept them safe by that name you gave me. None has been lost except the one doomed to destruction so that Scripture would be fulfilled"* (John 17:11-12). Jesus prays for protection over his disciples. This is a great example to us that when we pray for others we should pray for protection. Remember, at the time of this prayer Jesus is only hours away from leaving this earth to go back to his Father in heaven. He has been with his disciples and has protected them, now he prays that they will continue to be protected after he leaves. He then includes the one person who chose not to stay protected – Judas Iscariot, the traitor. Other than him, no one else was lost. The security we have in Jesus is eternal. And like Jesus, we can speak directly to our Father in heaven about anything. I would suggest that you ask God to protect your loved ones, your friends. I pray regularly for protection over my children, over my wife, and over those in my church. When I pray for protection, I pray specifically that God will lead them not into temptation but deliver them from the evil one, just as Jesus taught us to pray. Jesus prays this same thing for his disciples in verse 15 of John 17: *"My prayer is not that you take them out of the world but that you protect them from the evil one."*

The second thing Jesus prays is for his disciples to be sanctified (verse 17). This word means to become holy, to become like Jesus Christ. This should be something you pray for those you care about. The main thing should always remain the main thing, and the main thing is to experience salvation in all its fullness by becoming more like Jesus Christ every day. The Bible says that when we place our faith in Jesus Christ, we become a new person. This new person has to learn how to walk and then run. This is part of the sanctification process. As we submit to God's Spirit, we can become more like the one who gave us his Spirit. When we fight against God's Spirit, we stop growing. It is only through submission that one can grow. Salvation is easy – all we have to do is believe. Sanctification is hard because surrendering to God's will is a daily battle. I encourage you to pray that those you want to help would be sanctified, because this is the only way to realize who he or she truly has become. As I mentioned earlier, the purpose statement for our church is: To Develop Fully Devoted Followers of Christ. Pray this for those you love. Pray that they will be sanctified by God's Spirit to become all they are meant to be – fully devoted to Jesus. But don't expect others to become fully devoted if you are not fully devoted. You must be what you expect others to be. Pray for those you love, as you would want them to see you.

The last two things Jesus prays for are Unity and Knowledge (verses 20-25). He makes a shift in his prayer at this point. Instead of only praying for his disciples who were with him then, he prays for those who will become disciples through believing in his message later. He prays for you and for me! He prays first that we would experience unity. Notice, he did not pray for uniformity. Uniformity is like everyone marching in sync with the exact same movements and same uniform. Unity is not uniformity. Unity means that we are all heading in the same direction, but not necessarily with the same movements or uniform. Unity does not mean that we all march the same exact way, it doesn't mean that we look the same, and it also doesn't mean we dress the same. Unity is oneness expressed through diversity. In other words, for a team to be unified, it must have the same purpose. It must be heading in the same direction. Winning teams have unity. Jesus' disciples were unified because they all followed Christ; they were all heading in the same direction. In order to heal, you must also be heading in the same direction together. Those you hang out with should want to head in the same direction, otherwise you will get off track. Healing Steps have to move forward. This is why Jesus prayed that we would experience unity, because he knows that if not we will get off the path and head in the wrong direction. Unity is important;

not only in your healing, but also for those you love. Pray that they will experience the unity that only God's Spirit can bring through a union with Christ alone.

Knowledge is the last thing Jesus prays for. *"Righteous Father, though the world does not know you, I know you, and they know that you have sent me. I have made you known to them, and will continue to make you known in order that the love you have for me may be in them and that I myself may be in them"* (John 17:25-26). Why is knowledge important? Jesus said that if someone knows the truth, the truth would set him free. He also said that he is the truth (John 14:6). Truth is what is important about knowledge. Someone can know a lot of things, but if they don't know the truth, they are what the Bible calls foolish. Knowledge in itself is meaningless unless the knowledge leads somewhere – hopefully to the truth.

Notice what aspects of knowledge Jesus prays. He prays that even though those in the world do not know God, the ones who are In Christ know God because they know Christ. In fact, Jesus said that he came to make God known. This is so important to your faith and to your healing. The only way you can heal and grow in Christ is to know God, and the only way to know God is to know Christ. This is what you should pray for those you are trying to help. Pray that they will come to know Christ so that they can know God. When someone knows Christ, they know the truth because he is the truth! But knowledge is not the end goal, love is. Jesus prays that he made his Father known to us not so that we can know a lot about God, but so that we can know God's love. When you know God's truth, you will know God's love because the Bible says that God is love! Pray that those you love will know God's love.

Carry Them

"Where have you been?" The mother demanded. The little girl replied, "On my way home, I met a friend who was crying because she had broken her doll." "Oh," said her mother, "then you stopped to help her fix the doll?" "Oh, no," replied the little girl, "I stopped to help her cry." Sometimes prayers aren't enough.

During the three years of my battle with depression and physical illness, I would be comforted knowing people were praying for me. But what really helped me get through this time were those who stopped by to visit. Sometimes they would come and just sit with me. I remember one person sat with me for most of the day. It was amazing to see the outpouring of love and support that came my way.

I don't know about you, but I struggle with certain thoughts. Thoughts that tell me, "you don't deserve to be loved." These thoughts cause me to think that I am alone; that no one cares. This is not true. When people pray for me and love me by putting feet to their prayers, it shows me that I am loved. This does not change, however, the thoughts that tell me otherwise.

When I left my weeklong rehab experience, I was introduced to a man who became my sponsor. A sponsor is someone who leads and guides you through the steps of recovery. This person becomes someone who you count on, and who holds you to account. I remember when he gave me his phone number and told me to call him anytime. I asked, "what if it is 4:00 in the morning, can I call you then?" He answered, "Yes, anytime." Then he said something to me that I will never forget. He said, "David, what you don't understand is that I get as much out of helping you as you get out of receiving my help." Wow! These words rocked my world. I always thought the opposite. I always thought that when I requested help, it was a burden rather than a blessing. I felt like I was interrupting their schedule, but what I did not know is for many people, especially people who have come out the other end, helping others heal brings purpose to their life. This is how I see it now. I see helping others not as a burden, but as a blessing. Yes, helping others takes time and energy, but seeing someone "get it" brings me joy.

One main reason the Church exists it to help others heal. The Church should not be a museum for saints; the Church should be a hospital for sinners. Jesus said that he came for the sick and for the lost. In fact, he said that it is the sick that need a doctor. We are all to some degree sick. Thank God that he has healed us spiritually through faith in Christ. But, this does not change our prevalence to sickness. I still struggle with old habits, hurts and hang-ups. When someone says something to me that may come off as criticism, I automatically jump into "defensive" mode. This mode causes me to shut down and become argumentative and belligerent. The fact that I know this is reason to celebrate, because knowing something helps with diagnosing the problem. But knowing information is not enough to heal, one must relinquish control to God's Spirit. This is important because God is the only one who can heal you from the inside out.

One of the ways God heals is through others. We can see this through the health care industry. Finding a doctor who can help is key to ridding us of many physical diseases. However, what about spiritual diseases? Who helps us with those? The answer is that God can help us rid of spiritual sickness, and sometimes he chooses to work through the church. The Apostle Paul speaks of this in his letters to the church. He speaks of the importance of not just seeing our faith as individualistic and personal. He exhorts those who are in the church to see their faith also as a corporate affair. He speaks of individual believers as part of a whole, the Body of Christ. The Church is not about one person – except Jesus Christ. The Church is about each person coming together to form one body under the headship of Christ. When we function in this way, the body is healthy.

Paul wrote a letter to the Church in Galatia. He spends the first part of his letter reminding the believers there about who they are in Christ. What has happened to them because of their faith in Christ? But then he spends the latter part of the letter speaking of how to live out this new faith. It is not enough to just know information, it is more important to experience transformation. Transformation happens when you live by how God designed you to live. God has designed those who belong to Christ to live in community. This community is the Church. This is why it is so important for you to get plugged into a local Bible-believing and teaching church. You will experience healing when you are plugged into the healer – Jesus Christ – not only personally, but also corporately.

In chapter 6 of Galatians, Paul speaks of the importance of helping others heal. He says it this way: *"Brothers and sisters, if someone is caught in a sin, you who live by the Spirit should restore that person gently. But watch yourselves, or you also may be tempted. Carry each other's burdens, and in this way you will fulfill the law of Christ"* (Galatians 6:1-2). Look at how beautiful a statement this is. Paul does not deny that people in the church will sin. In fact, he expects that people will sin. But what he says to do, how he says to handle this, is exactly how the church should respond when a brother or sister in Christ falls.

First, he speaks of someone being caught in a sin. The word "caught" can mean to "overtake." This sentence could read, "Brothers and Sisters, if someone is *overtaken* by sin…" Isn't that beautiful? Not that someone sins, but the fact that God knows that sometimes we can't help it. Sometimes, no matter how much we try to do the right thing, sin overtakes us. But what does God say to do with someone like this? Does he say to kick this person out of the church? Well, sometimes he does say this, but only for those who are not willing to admit their problem. People who will not admit, cannot experience healing, and will also bring problems not only on themselves, but also on the entire church. Sin is like cancer. If someone has cancer, usually they will want to be healed of it. Some people, however, will not admit that they have cancer (sin) and, therefore, they cannot be healed. But when someone is willing to admit, then healing can begin. How does God say to deal with someone who is overtaken by sin? He tells those who are living by the Spirit (those who are well) to help the sick person (the one who sinned) be restored, but gently. The word "restored" can mean to "repair" or in medical terms, "restore a broken bone." When I was young, I broke my wrist. In order for my wrist to heal, the doctor had to reset the bone and then put it in a cast so that it would heal. This is how we are to help someone who has been overtaken by sin and willing to admit so. Those who are well are supposed to help those who are sick. This is how we are called to help others heal.

Notice, though, Paul gives a caution: "But watch yourselves!" There is a saying that goes, "you will become like who you hang out with." I remember a guy one time came to me and with glee said, "Pastor, I have found my calling. I am called to minister to strippers!" My first response was, "Lord, why wasn't that my calling?" I'm just kidding. That was not my response! My response was, "are you sure?" I mean, this guy turned out to be a recovering sex addict. That was not what God told him to do; this was something he just wanted to do. Someone's calling comes from God, not from our own made-up dreamland. The point is this: <u>Make sure that when you are helping someone heal, that you don't fall into the same trap and be overtaken as well</u>! That is what Paul means by his statement of caution. This means that you, even if you are well, need to make sure that you have other "well" people around you to hold you to account. There is a reason why Jesus sent out his disciples as missionaries paired in twos. When we try to help people without someone else keeping us accountable, we will inevitably fall and be overtaken. This is why we have to watch ourselves and allow others to watch as well.

Paul then makes this important statement: "Carry each other's burdens." The word carry is in the imperative form, which means this is a command. God is commanding the church in Galatia to do something that they may have not wanted to do. Sometimes the church can become a holy huddle where people gather in cliques and never see beyond themselves. This is not how the church should function. Since the church is a body, the church should be concerned about other body parts, even parts that are different than you. When someone is overtaken by sin, the last thing they need is to be judged. Now, again, this does not mean that we should not judge sin. We should judge sin. But we should start by judging our own sin! When we are able and willing to judge our own sin, then we can be a part of judging other sin. But when someone is overtaken and comes in humility and willing to admit, then those who are well, should help them heal and be restored by carrying them. After all, isn't that what Jesus has done for you?

I am not a tall man. So when my children were young, we would go to Disneyland and wait until the nighttime electrical parade. I would make sure I would stand as close to the action as possible. But there always seemed to be people in front of me blocking the view. I would pick up my child and put him on my shoulders. I wanted them to at least be able to see the parade, even if I could not. When someone is overtaken by sin, we should carry him or her so that they can see a path to healing and see their need for a Savior. Carrying someone takes sacrifice; it takes energy, it takes time. People don't usually become well overnight. The word "carry" can also mean "bear." Jesus carried his cross for us. His cross was very heavy. He bore the weight of his cross for us. Carrying someone is a heavy burden sometimes. When we pray for others, we can feel the pain somewhat; but when we get in the dirt with them, and see just how much they have been overtaken, the burden becomes almost unfathomable. We will cry with them, we will hurt with them, but in the end, we will rejoice as our Healer, God, works through us to help someone heal. There aren't a lot of experiences like seeing someone heal from being overtaken!

The Hole In The Roof

One day as Jesus was teaching in a house, a large crowd gathered. The crowd was so large that there was standing room only. Some men heard of this gathering and decided to take their friend to be healed. There was one problem, however, the friend was paralyzed and could not walk. These were days when wheelchairs had not existed so the friends had to carry their friend on a mat. When they got to the house, they could not enter due to the size of the crowd. So they did the unimaginable. They carried their friend to the top of the roof, and lowered him through a hole, and placed him right in front of Jesus.

Talk about tenacity! They were so dead set on carrying their friend to Jesus that nothing would stop them.

I have met people who will stop at nothing to bring their friends and loved ones to Jesus. They pray non-stop, they do everything they can, because they know that without Jesus, their friend will perish. I have met people who have not stopped inviting their friends to church because they know that Jesus is there. They will stop at nothing. Some people even drive miles out of their way to make sure their friend is placed before Jesus.

When we started The Gate Christian Bible Church, we were meeting in a school. Every Sunday, I would pick the church van up with all the equipment and drive it to the school where volunteers would meet to help set up the church. I found out that a relative of mine was living close to where we were meeting. This particular relative had been overtaken by alcohol, to the point of homelessness. He also happened to be very strong and big, and I knew I could use him to help with set up. I reached out to him and asked, but his response was that he was not interested in church. I asked again, saying that if he did not want to stay for the church service, that was fine, but at least would he help me with setting up. He agreed. I drove to his house early before church and knocked at the door, but he did not answer. He stood me up. I called him again, because I knew that the only way he was going to get well, was to be placed in front of Jesus. Finally, after a few tries, he came with me. He didn't come alone. He brought along with him a bota bag filled with vodka. And this was 7:00 in the morning! He helped me set up, but did not stay. He took the bus home. For weeks, I picked him up, and for weeks, he would show up with his vodka and take the bus home. Finally, he decided to stay for church. There he was, in church, he and his vodka. No one judged him. In fact we loved on him. The day his life changed was a day when he finally admitted his sickness. He gave his life to Jesus Christ, and I had the privilege and honor of baptizing him. To this day, over ten years later, he is sober and married. He realizes that if it were not for Jesus, he would be dead.

I share this story to show that sometimes it takes multiple attempts of taking someone to Jesus. You may have to make a hole in the roof, but don't give up! You never know when your effort will pay off. I think people give up way too early. These guys who dropped their friend off at Jesus' feet went to great effort, but it paid off. The Bible says that when Jesus saw their faith, he healed the man right there in front of them. The man got up and walked home! Notice the pronoun "their." Jesus did not just acknowledge the paralyzed man's faith; he acknowledged the faith of his friends to stop at nothing to bring him to Jesus. God honors this kind of faith. They carried their friend to Jesus and their friend was healed. This is the kind of faith I want you to have. This is the kind of faith that moves mountains. Don't give up! Your miracle might be just around the corner.

<u>Invite Them</u>

When I was young and an aspiring musician, I looked forward to being around influential people. My hope was that I would meet someone who would open the door to attaining a record deal. I was around sixteen years old at the time when my friend John met a very influential record producer. John shared with him about our band. The next thing I know, we were being invited to come to his house in the Hollywood Hills to record. He told John that he was going to record us on 8-track. I was so excited because I had never recorded in a professional studio before. We arrived at his house to find out that he was not recording us on an 8-track professional recorder; he was going to record us on an 8-track cassette tape. You might not even know what an 8-track cassette looks like. These were nothing more than glorified cassette tapes. Nevertheless, the fact that we were invited to this producer's home to record was something to brag about, especially since this record producer went on to discover and record Rick Springfield!

The point of that story is that we all have a desire to be invited to something important. This is why it is so amazing that Jesus Christ would invite people to follow him. "Follow me," he would say. Some accepted and others declined. Isn't it amazing that people decline an invitation from God himself? Do you know that Jesus has invited you? He has invited you to come to him. He says, *"Come to me all who are tired and I will give you rest"* (Matthew 11:28). Jesus invites you to a place of rest. If you are tired of trying to control everything, if you are tired of trying to run the show, then come to Jesus. You will feel a whole lot better! He offers rest to those who are tired, burdened, and weary. He offers life that is everlasting and power that is supernatural. He offers peace that goes well beyond our understanding of peace, at least with regards to the kind of peace the world offers. God's peace is transcendent beyond circumstances, because God's peace is not reliant on circumstances. God's peace is a heavenly peace that only he can give.

Since Jesus has gone out of his way to invite you, shouldn't you also go out of your way to invite others to come to Christ? Inviting someone to come to Christ is easy. Yet we become uneasy and fearful because we are more concerned about their response than our invitation. I remember shortly after I came to Christ how God challenged me to invite people and how I wilted in fear. One particular time was filled with embarrassment. There I was in the men's public restroom. As I was doing what we do in the restroom, the Lord put on my heart to tell the man next to me that Jesus loves him. "Are you kidding God? Now?" Needless to say, I did not invite that man to come to Christ! Another time was when I was fueling up my car at the gas station. The button on the fuel pump said, "Push if you need assistance." I heard the Lord say to me, "push the button and tell the man inside that Jesus loves him." Again, I argued and debated with God and drove away without pushing the button. Why is this? It is because I was more concerned about what the other person would think of me than about the other person missing God's invitation. Now, sometimes we can beat ourselves up for not inviting people. Don't do that. But learn from your mistakes. Trust God. Yes, God does not need us to invite people; he can do it on his own. In fact, God does not need anything, yet he includes us. But when we miss inviting others to come to Christ for healing, it is us who miss the blessing of leading others to Christ. There is nothing that feels the same as leading someone to Christ. Remember, God has healed you, not so you will just experience your healing for yourself, but that you will help others heal by inviting them to come to Christ.

Teach Them

Moments before Jesus ascended to his Father after he was raised from the dead, he spoke to his disciples. What he said is documented in the Bible in Matthew chapter 28. In the very last documented word written in Matthew's gospel, Jesus commands his disciples to do certain things. He told them the following three commands: (1)

Make disciples; (2) Baptize them; (3) Teach them. Let's look briefly at these three commands.

"Go therefore and make disciples of all nations" (Matthew 28:19). Some people think this means that you have to go somewhere other than where you are. This is not true. This word means to make disciples as you go. This does not mean that I have to travel to a distant land; I can stay right where I am. This is good news, because I have lived other places. There is no weather like southern California weather. I have lived in Texas, and I have to tell you, I am glad I live where I live. Nevertheless the command to make disciples is not something that is an option, it is imperative. A disciple is someone who is a student, a learner. Remember, Disciples of Christ are students of Christ. A student of Jesus Christ studies hard to be found faithful. This means that a disciple of Jesus Christ does what Jesus Christ says to do. Our job is to help others heal by making them into disciples. This is hard work, but it is important work. This is not someone else's job it is your job. Are you making disciples? If not, why not?

The second thing Jesus tells us is to baptize the disciples you reach in the name of the Father, the Son, and the Holy Spirit. Water baptism is the sign of a believer. It is similar to my wedding ring. My wedding ring does not make me married; it is a symbol of my marriage. The ring is an outward expression of an inward commitment and love. Water baptism is an outward sign of an inward commitment and love for Jesus Christ. Water baptism does not save you, because we are saved by grace, but water baptism should be the first act of obedience for someone who comes to Christ in faith.

The third command Jesus gives us in this passage is to teach those who we reach to obey everything God has taught us. When we help others heal, we must remember that healing comes by way of the Word of God, along with His Spirit working in someone's life. Jesus said that the truth would set us free. When we know the truth, we will be truly free. Freedom is a symptom of health. When someone is truly healed, they are truly free; no matter the circumstance, the truth is always written in the heart of the healed person. God tells us that he will write his commands on our heart and put his Spirit in us; therefore, we have everything we need to live a healed life. Helping others heal is helping them learn the commands of God and holding them accountable to stay on the path. When we love someone and we see this person veering off the path, we must tell him. This is the responsibility of the teacher. We are all teachers because we are all disciples. From one disciple to the next, let's keep each other on the path and carry each other if one of us is overtaken by sin.

Congratulations, you have finished the last step on the path to healing. Healing Steps, the A, B, C's of healing begin the moment you **A**dmit you have a problem that you can't solve on your own. You then **B**elieve that God can solve your problem and give you the help you need. You must **C**ommit your life and will over to the care of God and **D**iscuss your problems with God and with other people. **E**mbrace God's will for your life by **F**orgiving those who have hurt you and learning to forgive yourself. Continue on the path to healing by **G**rowing in your relationship with God and then **H**elping others heal. Those are the A, B, C's of healing. But knowing them is not enough. You must put them to practice. You must start to walk so that you can learn to run. Get involved with others and go through these steps together. Use the Stepping Stones workbook to help you delve deeper and start a Healing Steps ministry at your church.

I look forward to all that God has for you as you walk with him on the Path to Healing.

Works Cited:

AA Big Book. Alcoholics Anonymous World Services, 1939, 1955, 1976, 2001

Campbell, Mike; Henley, Donald H; Campbell Mike. The Heart Of The Matter. Sony/ATV Music Publishing LLC, Warner Chappell Music, Inc.

Courson, Jon. *Jon Courson's Application Commentary, New Testament*. Thomas Nelson, 2003.

Joel, Billy. *Piano Man*. Sony/ATV Music Publishing LLC, Universal Music Publishing Group.

Petty, Tom. *The Waiting*. Sony/ATV Music Publishing LLC, Warner/ Chappell Music, Inc.

Stanley, Charles. The Principle of the Path. Thomas Nelson, 2011

Stokes. Benton, Kevin. Wood, Tony W. *Sometimes He Calms The Storm*. Universal Music Publishing Group

Notes

Chapter 1

[1] Petty, Tom. *The Waiting*. (Sony/ATV Music Publishing LLC, Warner/Chappell Music, Inc.)

Chapter 3

[1] Stanley, Charles. The Principle of the Path. (Thomas Nelson 2011)

Chapter 5

[1] Richards Keith. Jaggger, Mick. *You Can't Always Get What You Want*. (Abkco Music, Inc.)

[2] Stokes. Benton, Kevin. Wood, Tony W. *Sometimes He Calms The Storm*. (Universal Music Publishing Group)

[3] *AA Big Book*. (Alcoholics Anonymous World Services, 1939, 1955, 1976, 2001)

Chapter 6

[1] Campbell, Mike; Henley, Donald H; Campbell Mike. *The Heart Of The Matter*. (Sony/ATV Music Publishing LLC, Warner Chappell Music, Inc.)

[2] Joel, Billy. *Piano Man*. (Sony/ATV Music Publishing LLC, Universal Music Publishing Group.)

[3] Courson, Jon. *Jon Courson's Application Commentary, New Testament*.)Thomas Nelson, 2003)

[4] *mb-soft.com* (accessed February 9, 2016)

Printed in the USA
CPSIA information can be obtained
at www.ICGtesting.com
JSHW011912030823
45865JS00002B/12